SLEEP
WELL
EVERY
NIGHT

Also by Glenn Harrold

De-stress Your Life
Lose Weight Now!
Look Young, Live Longer
The Answer

SLEEP
WELL
EVERY
NIGHT

**A new approach to getting
a good nights sleep**

Glenn Harrold

First published in Great Britain in 2008 by Orion Books
This edition first published in 2019 by Orion Spring
an imprint of The Orion Publishing Group Ltd
Carmelite House, 50 Victoria Embankment
London EC4Y 0DZ

An Hachette UK Company

1 3 5 7 9 10 8 6 4 2

Every effort has been made to ensure that the information in the book
is accurate. The information in this book may not be applicable in each
individual case so it is advised that professional medical advice is obtained
for specific health matters and before changing any medication or dosage.
Neither the publisher nor author accepts any legal responsibility for any
personal injury or other damage or loss arising from the use of the
information in this book. In addition, if you are concerned about
your diet or exercise regime and wish to change them, you
should consult a health practitioner first.

A CIP catalogue record for this book is
available from the British Library.

ISBN 978 1 4091 8556 7

Printed and bound in Great Britain by Clays Ltd, Elcograf, S.p.A.

I dedicate this book to my mum, who passed away while I was writing it. She was diagnosed with terminal cancer out of the blue and given days to live. She faced this challenge with immense courage and dignity, and that will always be a great inspiration to me. God bless you, Ma – you were something special.

CONTENTS

WELCOME

Congratulations! You have just taken the first step towards achieving good sleeping habits. *Sleep Well Every Night* is a unique sleep programme that is guaranteed to improve your sleep and give you more energy throughout the day. After following the steps in this book and listening to the accompanying hypnotherapy audio, you will feel less stressed, be able to fall asleep more easily and be less likely to wake during the night. Sleeping well will enable you to live your life free from tiredness and exhaustion. You will also feel healthier and be much more productive in your day-to-day activities.

Sleep deprivation is a form of torture, so don't feel bad if your moods have been up and down or you have felt grumpy, angry and frustrated at times. Sleeping problems are extremely common and can have many repercussions in your daily life. This book and audio (available to download online) will help you through this difficult time and help you rest your body and relax your mind in a completely safe, natural way. You have taken positive action and things are going to change for you.

Welcome to the rest of your life!

INTRODUCTION

Long ago, our ancestors would rise when it was light, work and play during daylight hours, wind down as the night approached, and sleep when it became dark. The only source of illumination after dark was fire. Consequently, they followed the natural rhythms of the sun, and probably slept very well because of it. You can bet your life the equivalent of insomnia didn't exist then.

Humans, along with most animals, are biologically hard-wired to sleep at the onset of darkness. We have been designed that way so that we can get the best from each day. So responsive are our bodies to differences in light and dark that our circadian rhythms, or internal biological clocks, are even programmed to reset with each change of season.

This worked well in the pre-industrial world, when our lifestyles were very much in sync with the natural rhythms of life. In the late-nineteenth century, however, when Thomas Edison invented the electric light bulb, everything changed. Since then, we have become increasingly out of balance with our biological clocks.

Even in the few hundred years before the advent of

electricity, it was only the elite few who could afford the luxury of burning candles late into the night, so the vast majority had no option but to take to their beds when it became dark. Even so, the natural light from candles is not enough to alter our internal biological clocks in the way that strong electric lighting does. It seems hard now to imagine the sun being our only source of illumination, but that was the case for the vast majority of our history. It is only in the last hundred or so years that we have had electricity in the home, which is a minuscule period of time if you think in terms of our evolution as a whole.

Now, in today's 24/7 world, we are able to watch TV at all hours, work late into the night and be entertained in a multitude of ways long after it gets dark. Shops and bars stay open all night in our 24-hour consumer-driven society. As a result of having so many night-time options, the importance of sleep has slowly been eroded. In our technologically advanced society, we are sleeping less than at any time in our history. It is estimated that nearly 50 per cent of people in the UK and US are sleep-deprived to some degree.

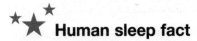

Human sleep fact

A hundred years ago, we slept on average for nine to ten hours a night – two hours more than we do today.

Our round-the-clock lifestyles are causing us major problems.

We once believed that technology would allow us to have more time on our hands, when in reality all it has done is make us busier than ever. The fact that we work longer, play harder and are more productive means we often sleep less than we should. We also face many diverse mental stresses and pressures, and have so many choices to make in an average day that it is said that we make more decisions in a week than our grandparents made in a year. Being overloaded with mental pressures can make it hard to switch off when we go to bed at night. It is no wonder that so many people have trouble sleeping.

A solution to many sleep problems lies in hypnosis, as it is a wonderful tool for quietening the mind and relaxing the body. Hypnosis has exactly the same effect on brainwave cycles as sleep. The transgression from full consciousness into a hypnotic trance will steadily slow your brainwaves and naturally guide you into a state that is ideal for deep, restful sleep. This winding-down process should happen automatically when you go to bed at night, but many people need a little help, and this book and audio could very well be your answer.

About me

Before becoming a hypnotherapist, I worked for many years as a musician. During my teens, in the distant 1970s, I was a punk rocker and played bass in a band that achieved a degree of success, which came and went like Halley's Comet. Later, when my son was born, I mellowed and binned my bondage trousers, dog collar and green hair, and proceeded to spend a number of years earning a living playing guitar in a covers duo. We sometimes played clubs where we shared the bill with stage hypnotists. Some of these shows were a little dodgy to say the least, but they did spark my interest in the subject. I had no desire to use hypnosis for entertainment – giving people suggestions that they would feel attracted to a broom or believe they were Elvis just wasn't my thing – but I became fascinated with hypnosis's potential to heal and transform.

I have always gained great personal satisfaction from helping people get over all kinds of stress-related problems, and in the early 1990s, I completed a two-year diploma with the London School of Clinical Hypnosis which gave me an excellent foundation. Since then I have treated thousands of clients in individual hypnotherapy sessions and have dealt with every kind of sleep problem. I have also helped people to achieve lifelong goals, lose weight, stop smoking, overcome fears and phobias, build their self-confidence and much more. There is no shortcut to experience and I have practised one-to-one hypnotherapy for many years. Then, after gaining invaluable grass-roots experience, I drew upon my musical background and began making hypnosis recordings, primarily to support my work with clients.

The combination of my hypnotherapy experience and production knowledge enabled me to make professional and effective recordings. I went on to sell them in many stores, and I started my own publishing company to market and distribute them. I had no experience of marketing or publishing, but simply used my self-hypnosis skills to help me succeed in business. At the time of writing, my hypnosis and meditation audios have sold nearly 10 million copies worldwide, and my CDs are still the UK's best-selling self-help CDs of all time. Via iTunes and other download sites, they have also become one of the world's most downloaded self-help series.

I believe they have sold so well because my aim was to create recordings that were genuinely effective and I put a lot of love and care into producing them. The feedback I get from people who buy them is amazing, and I feel genuinely privileged to be able to help others in this way.

I felt compelled to write this book and create an

accompanying recording because I know just how many people's lives are negatively affected by poor-quality sleep, and I know that hypnotherapy can make a genuine difference. My approach to overcoming sleep problems is tried and tested, simple and effective, and I want to share it with as many people as possible who are suffering with the debilitating problem of sleep deprivation. You really can change your sleeping habits if you are willing to follow these simple steps.

This book and the accompanying *Sleep Well* audio recording will provide you with the solution you need to sleep well every night. Listen to the audio each night and follow the Sleep Well Programme and you will be getting a good night's sleep in no time. Good-quality sleep is one of the main keys to health and longevity, and to slowing the ageing process, so it is vital that you follow the Sleep Well Programme. By doing this, you will recondition your mind to sleep well and soon this habit will feel completely natural. As a reminder of the most important points from the Sleep Well Programme, I have included seven Golden Sleep Rules. Follow these religiously and every night will be a good night's sleep.

How the book works

The book has three main sections. Section 1 looks into sleep and hypnosis in more detail, and also offers tips and techniques. Section 2 contains my unique Sleep Well Programme, which gives you the ultimate solution for almost all sleep problems and will help you establish healthy sleep patterns in a short space of time. Simply follow the six steps and you will free yourself from destructive sleeping patterns for ever. It is a completely safe approach and can help you achieve good sleep patterns without the unhealthy side-effects associated with long-term medication use. Drugs only ever treat the symptoms, whereas hypnotherapy is a natural solution that will help you overcome the root causes of your problem. Focus on the areas that are most relevant to your situation. If your biggest problem is that you struggle to switch off because of a busy mind, then give more attention to the techniques that help in this area.

Section 3 looks at some of the other key areas that can cause sleepless nights – chiefly anxiety, financial worries and even electromagnetic fields – and offers a number of techniques for combating these. I have also included information on creating a sleep diary and working out how much sleep you need. At the end of the book, there is a Further Resources section, which recommends books, CDs, DVDs and apps that may be of extra help to you, as well as some general information and contacts.

Sleep problems come in many different forms and will require different treatments, so throughout the book I have included a number of case studies in which people have overcome their sleep problems either by using my recordings or through working with me one-to-one. If any relate to your specific sleep problem, then the solution in these case studies may help to guide you in a certain direction.

When you start to use the self-hypnosis and visualisation techniques in this book, don't worry if you feel you're not doing them right or that not much has happened. The more you practise, the easier it becomes to switch off and go into a trance. Affirmations and visualisations are a remarkably effective reprogramming method, and even if it doesn't feel like it, they will make a big impact on your inner thought processes. Just closing your eyes, breathing deeply and really focusing on the affirmations as you say them will begin to make significant positive changes in the way you think and feel about your health and ability to sleep well.

Equally, don't worry about not going deep enough into a trance. The most important part of hypnosis is focusing your attention on a specific goal while you are relaxed and receptive to change. The keys to creating new positive patterns of behaviour are to believe the suggestions are reality and to put feeling into your affirmations as you repeat them. The more you feel them, the stronger the suggestions will anchor themselves in your unconscious.

You will be surprised at how effective affirmations can be in even the lightest of trances. The power of the unconscious mind works in a very subtle way. The most important things to remember are to enjoy the process and to have faith, because as with all things, the more you practise, the better you become!

How the audio download works

The *Sleep Well* audio download that accompanies this book can be downloaded for free, here: **www.glenn-harrold.com/orion/sleep**. It was created to still your mind and guide you into a deep, relaxing sleep. For maximum effect, I recommend you listen to the tracks through headphones while lying down, so that you can absorb all the positive suggestions and affirmations on a deeper level. I also suggest that you start using the audio programme as soon as possible because the hypnotherapy session will give you a great start. Once you feel you are in control and sleeping well, you can use the soundtrack as a back-up whenever you feel the need.

The audio download is completely safe, very effective and comes with a clear set of instructions. It is a full 30-minute hypnotherapy session, which you can use each night before you go to sleep. Just make sure you are careful not to get headphone leads caught round your neck when you listen in bed. You must on no account listen to the session while driving a vehicle or using heavy machinery. The recording will guide you into a state of complete physical and mental relaxation, so you must only listen while you are lying down in a place where you won't be disturbed.

Even if you fall asleep before you reach the end of the session, which will be mission accomplished in this case, you will still absorb all the positive suggestions up to the point that you went into a deep, somnambulistic state.

How long should I use the audio download for?

There are no hard and fast rules as to how long the session should be used, as it will work differently for each individual. It is impossible to give an estimated time for use, but after listening a few times you should begin to notice some positive changes. For some people, the positive changes will be instant and dramatic, and you will be guided to sleep every time you use it. Others may experience a gradual, subtle progression into improved sleep patterns. For maximum effect, listen every night until you feel you have achieved your aim and the new sleep patterns have become a habit. You can continue listening even after you have established good sleeping habits, as this will reinforce them.

Affirmations and sound effects on the audio

There are four stages of the *Sleep Well* audio download: the introduction, the induction, the trance deepening and the post-hypnotic suggestions and affirmations. On other titles, like *De-stress Your Life*, there is an additional fifth stage, the awakening, which brings the listener back to full waking consciousness. As the aim is to guide you to sleep and keep you there, this is not used on the *Sleep Well* audio.

The first thing you will hear is the introductory music and an explanation of how it works. After a few minutes, the music fades and you are left with a pleasant voice and some uniquely created sound effects, which will guide you into a state of complete physical and mental relaxation. The subtle sound effects have been carefully developed for maximum impact. Some of them have been recorded at 60 beats per minute to help synchronise the left and right hemispheres of the brain and create a very receptive learning state. The sounds are also recorded in certain keys and at frequencies that induce feelings of relaxation.

In addition to using your feelings and emotions, the other key to absorbing hypnotic suggestion is compoun-ding. This means that the more you hear the suggestions on the audio track and use the self-hypnosis techniques in this book, the quicker your unconscious mind will get the message. You will then respond to the suggestions automatically when you go to bed each night.

For more information on how to use the hypno-therapy audio download, please visit the Frequently Asked Questions page on the website www.hypno-sisaudio.com.

SECTION 1

UNDERSTANDING
SLEEP
AND THE
POWER OF HYPNOSIS

Chapter 1

WHAT IS SLEEP?

It's amazing to think that we spend a third of our lives asleep and yet no one really knows exactly what happens when we sleep or when we dream. There are many different convincing theories, but none that everyone agrees on.

Sleep is a mental and physical resting state in which we are relatively inactive and unaware of the outside world. When we sleep, we enter a world of our own, one that we have little control over, unlike when we are awake and controlling our thoughts and feelings consciously. Sleep is an experience that we cannot share with others. It's a personal journey into the world of the unconscious, which is why it's so hard to define.

We know that a good night's sleep allows our mind and body to rest so that they can re-energise and rejuvenate. One theory of what happens while we are asleep is that our brain performs vital housekeeping tasks, such as absorbing information; this could be in the form of assimilating things we have learned or storing memories of the day's events. Another theory is that sleep allows the unconscious mind to store new information and organise past, present and future thoughts and feelings. We know for certain that sleep has a major impact on brain development, as it affects cognitive skills such as thinking, speech and memory. Without regular healthy sleep, these skills become impaired.

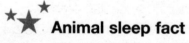 **Animal sleep fact**

Most species of primate, like chimps, monkeys and baboons, sleep on average for ten hours a day. However, the sleepiest primate is the owl monkey, which requires 17 hours' sleep a day in order to avoid being grumpy and irritable.

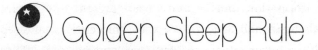# Golden Sleep Rule

1. Create a sleep diary.

Get in the habit of going to bed at the same time every night, even at weekends. This will help you regulate your sleep patterns, meaning you should wake up at the same time each morning and become sleepy at the same time each evening.

The length of your sleep will depend on how much rest your body requires. Keeping a regular sleep diary is the first step to conditioning your mind and body to go to sleep at the same time each night. See page 164 for how to start a sleep diary.

Circadian rhythms

Circadian rhythms, which form our internal biological clock, are the main reason why we sleep. Physiological functions that are circadian include most bodily functions, body temperature, hormone levels and digestion. The most obvious circadian rhythm is the cycle of sleep and wakefulness that repeats over a 24-hour period. So it is that humans have a natural cycle of approximately the length of one day – which is quite handy if you think about it!

Small structures in the brain control our circadian rhythms, and these respond to the presence or absence of light. This is one reason why daytime sleep has been found to be less restful than night-time sleep. We are simply not designed to sleep in the daytime. Our circadian rhythms are programmed to put us to sleep when it is dark and to wake us from the onset of daylight. However, studies have shown that the absence of light does not disable our biological clocks, so even if we stay awake all night and sleep in the day for long periods of time, our body is still programmed to sleep at night. This is why problems occur if we disrupt our natural sleep cycles; we are going against our in-built biological programme.

It has been shown that even plants have these fixed

☽ Sleep tip – daylight refresher

When you wake up, expose yourself to the daylight as soon as possible, as this will help to regulate your body's natural biological clock. If you can also include a short exercise workout in the daylight as soon as you wake, you will start the day in the best possible way.

internal rhythms. Studies have demonstrated that when plants display their opening and closing-up processes when daylight and darkness occur, these rhythms continue even when they are placed in environments in which there is no cycle of dark and light.

Although our biological clocks are programmed to run over a 24-hour period, they also respond to environmental time cues so that they remain in synchronicity with the physical world. Light is the main cue for resetting and synchronising our biological clock. The reason for this is because the length of daylight changes with the seasons. Our internal clocks automatically adjust with the

❝Not until just before dawn do people sleep best; not until people get old do they become wise.❞

Chinese proverb

☽ Sleep tip – valuing your sleep

Get into the habit of thinking of all the benefits you get from a good night's sleep. At eight o'clock every night, start to think about going to sleep and begin to look forward to being tucked up in your warm bed in the darkness. If you do this every night, you will start to value your sleep and see it as an important part of your day, which of course it is.

seasons to remain in sync. This amazing feat of human engineering also occurs in animals, enabling them to adjust to the seasons and get the most from their natural environment. When you learn these things, you realise we are designed to adapt to our environment perfectly.

Circadian rhythms follow a daily pattern. For most people, sleepy peaks occur every 12 hours: in the early hours of the morning and around mid-afternoon. The mid-afternoon dip is called a post-prandial dip and is caused by a natural decrease in body temperature. When our body temperature begins to drop, we are sleepier than when it begins to rise.

When you are aware of your body's natural dips

and highs, you can use this information to get the best out of your day. For example, if you are particularly prone to a post-prandial dip at 3 p.m. each day, try to avoid important meetings or anything that requires extra mental or physical effort at that time. Not always possible, I know, but when you have the option to schedule your day, avoiding natural dips will help you to use your energy more effectively.

If your sleep patterns are out of sync, perhaps because of jet lag caused by travelling through time zones or simply because of too many late nights, this disruption will affect when your daily highs and lows occur. However, it is something you can remedy quickly by re-establishing a good routine of sleep. Because your biological rhythms are hard-wired, it is simply a matter of getting back in sync with them. Imagine a surfer riding waves; every now and again he will fall off his surfboard halfway through the wave cycle, but he then gets back into the groove, rides out the next wave cycle perfectly and is back in sync.

Unless you have the most predictable of routines and few demands on your time, there will always be occasions when your sleep patterns get disrupted and you are out of sync with your natural body clock. When this happens, just make an extra effort to get back into a good sleep routine as soon as possible. Getting the right balance is the key to most things in life.

Why is sleep so important?

It is said that human beings gravitate towards pleasure. In psychology, there is a term called delayed gratification, which is linked to intelligence and describes the ability to put off an immediate gratification for a bigger reward later on. In this day and age, there are many distractions and temptations that keep us from our beds at night. We often opt for the instant fix of staying up late to watch TV instead of going to bed early with the rewards that

☽ Sleep tip – the warm bath

A warm bath an hour or so before bedtime will help you to prepare for sleep. Not only does it encourage you to relax and unwind, but it also temporarily raises your body temperature. After getting out of the bath, your body temperature will slowly cool down, creating the ideal physiological state for sleep.

Make sure the water is comfortably warm but not too hot, and don't spend more than 20 minutes in the bath.

will bring the next day. Even though we know staying up late at night will make us feel groggy the next day, we often succumb to this temptation because sleep is given so little importance in our lives.

Sleep is a vital biological function and is essential to our physical and emotional well-being. The body produces chemicals like melatonin to help us achieve good-quality, deep sleep. Melatonin is a hormone created by the pineal gland, which is a small ball of nerve cells that are located between the two hemispheres of the brain. The pineal gland responds to light and darkness, and only when it is dark does it release the melatonin that induces sleep. This is why sleeping in complete darkness is so important. It is also interesting to note that we produce more melatonin in the winter months, when the nights are darker for longer. This again shows that we are synchronised to adapt to the natural rhythms of our external world.

When we sleep well, we wake feeling refreshed and energised with a clear mind. This is because we have produced enough melatonin and have rested our brain and body for the right amount of time. When you stay up too late or have a night of disturbed sleep,

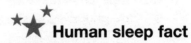 **Human sleep fact**

Babies sleep for about 17 hours a day – just over two-thirds of their day.

★ Human sleep fact

For the average adult aged between 25 and 55, eight hours' sleep a night is considered optimal. Small children and teenagers need about ten hours' sleep a night, while people over 65 need about six hours.

you are all too aware of the after-effects. The next day, you feel drowsy, lethargic, forgetful, irritable, foggy-headed and lacking in energy and clarity of thought. Also affected is the part of the brain that controls language, memory, planning and sense of time. This is because lack of sleep affects the brain's ability to recuperate and recharge. It affects cognitive functioning and emotional and physical health, and in some cases can be linked to depression.

We can go to sleep when we sit up, perhaps on an aeroplane, a train or catnapping at a desk, but the quality of sleep will not be good. This is because when you are upright, as soon as you nod off your muscles relax, you begin to sway, and the defence mechanism in your brain wakes you up. This happens as soon as you descend beyond the light stage of sleep into the deeper stages of sleep, so sleeping sitting up does not allow you to achieve the deeper restorative sleep that is needed to recharge. Some animals are designed to sleep while sitting up, but not humans. To get quality sleep, we must always lie down.

Quality and quantity of sleep are equally important.

We need on average between six and eight hours' sleep a night. Some people can function well on four or five hours; others will need nine or ten. The amount we need can also vary from night to night, depending on the kind of day we have had. If you have spent the day exerting a lot of physical energy, engaging in many different conversations or dealing with stressful situations, you may need more sleep that night than if you have had a quiet day with few demands on your brain and body.

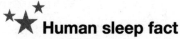

Human sleep fact

To sleep, our body temperature needs to drop, which is one reason why hot summer nights can cause restless sleep.

Poor-quality sleep happens when the sleep is disturbed or not deep enough to reach the deepest sleep state so that restorative changes can take place. In the next chapter, we'll look at what effect this has on your mind and body.

What happens when we sleep?

When we sleep, we experience a general decrease in body temperature, blood pressure, breathing rate and most other bodily functions. In contrast, the human brain never decreases in activity: studies have shown that the brain is as active during sleep as it is when awake. Having said that, when we sleep, our conscious, analytical thought processes stop, but our unconscious thoughts continue. This is why we often have dreams that make no logical sense – our logical thinking is switched off and unable to make sense of the dream. When we wake, our conscious, analytical thought processes are restored. If we recall the events in the dream, we then naturally try to form them in a logical order in an attempt to understand them. It is wonderful that we can't always understand our dreams, as it would be a boring world if we had all the answers. The unconscious processes of sleep and dreaming are two of the great mysteries of life.

In psychology, our conscious and unconscious thought processes are explained by the iceberg analogy – the conscious, analytical part of our mind is the 10 per cent of the iceberg above the water; the unconscious part is the 90 per cent

★★ **Human sleep fact**

Snoring only occurs in non-REM sleep.

that is submerged. As we go to sleep, our conscious mind slowly switches off, allowing us direct access to our unconscious. The unconscious mind is the part where our innermost fears and anxieties lie. It is also where our creativity and talents are to be found. This is why we sometimes wake up with great ideas or fearful thoughts. When this happens, your unconscious mind has been processing information while you were asleep; when you wake, this filters through to your conscious thoughts. This information can be confusing and difficult to make sense of, but your feelings will always tell you if you have experienced something positive or negative while you were asleep.

When we sleep, our brainwaves slow down and nerve cells in our brain synchronise their electrical activity. Electrodes placed on the scalp can detect those brain patterns that characterise the sleep state. It is not true that we go from being awake and pass through deeper and deeper states of sleep until we wake. Sleep is a cyclical process; we go through various cycles of light and deep sleep throughout the night.

During an eight-hour sleep cycle, we alternate between two different sleep states: non-REM (non-rapid eye movement) and REM. Throughout non-REM sleep, muscle activity is still functional,

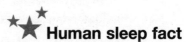

Human sleep fact

Premature babies require more REM sleep than babies born on time.

★ ★ Human sleep fact

We tend to dream less as we get older.

breathing is low, and brain activity is minimal. It consists of four stages that gradually deepen from light to deep sleep. The REM sleep state that follows is deeper still and is characterised by rapid eye movement, in which the eyeballs move around beneath the eyelids. This also occurs with subjects in hypnosis, and it serves as a good indicator to the hypnotherapist that the subject is in a deep hypnotic trance.

A typical night of sleep begins with about 80 minutes of four-stage light to deep non-REM sleep, followed by an REM period of about ten minutes. (This 90-minute cycle in adult sleep lasts for 60 minutes for infants.) The cycle occurs four to five times a night. Approximately 75 per cent of the first sleep cycle is spent in non-REM sleep. In the successive cycles through the night, the proportion of the cycle occupied by REM sleep tends to increase. It seems that non-REM dominates the early part of the night and REM the early-morning part just before waking.

Most dreaming takes place during REM sleep; it does occur in non-REM sleep but to a significantly lesser extent. It is possible that we dream constantly through-out all sleep cycles, though the dreams will vary in intensity. The deeper REM dreams are more surreal, more visual and stronger in feeling and depth, but in the lighter non-REM state, dreams are less intense and more logical. The reason for this may be that when you are in a non-REM state of consciousness, you are using more of your logical thought processes, as defined by the iceberg analogy earlier. When you are in REM sleep, much like deep hypnosis you are using a greater part of your unconscious mind.

Fluttering eyelids, muscle paralysis, irregular breathing and increased heart rate and blood pressure occur during REM sleep, and these physiological responses further distinguish it from the non-REM state. REM sleep is also called paradoxical sleep because brainwave activity is similar to an awakened state. It is during REM sleep that the brain sends signals to the muscles to remain immobile so dreams will not be acted out.

★ Animal sleep fact

In common with humans, dolphins are warm-blooded mammals that need to breathe air. They would drown if they fell asleep underwater. Consequently, they have evolved so that when they sleep, only one half of their brain switches off, while the other remains awake. The two halves of their brain then alternate roles every few hours. This is called unihemispheric sleep. Many birds are also hard-wired for unihemispheric sleep so that they can remain vigilant against predators.

The hidden observer

Part of the mind remains awake even when we are in an unconscious state, studies have shown. This part of the mind has been called the hidden observer and has been described as a cognitive error-detection system that can alert us to an external danger when we are in an unconscious state. So if you were asleep and there was danger around you, the hidden observer would alert you and bring you back to full consciousness very quickly.

A strong characteristic of sleep is the reduction in responsiveness to sight, sound and smell, but although we achieve sensory isolation when we sleep, it is highly selective. For example, we can sleep through familiar loud noises like busy traffic that we are conditioned to hearing, but quieter, unfamiliar noise may wake us quickly.

A friend of mine once told me that he awoke suddenly one night to find an intruder entering his bedroom with a weapon. He had heard no sound and is a very heavy sleeper, but the air of impending danger was enough to wake him instantly from his deep sleep. He then made a lot of noise and scared the intruder into a retreat. It is nice to think that his hidden observer saved him that night.

The existence of the hidden observer has divided the scientific community, but stories like this go a long way towards demonstrating that we have an in-built warning mechanism that alerts us to danger even as we sleep.

☯ The unconscious mind case study

Not long ago I saw a gentleman who would fall asleep quite easily but wake every night at 3 a.m. almost to the second. Over a few sessions I regressed him back to the cause of his problem, which was outside of his conscious awareness. During the regression he went back to an incident that occurred at boarding school, some 50 years previously. At this point, he became quite emotional and had a full-blown abreaction. An abreaction allows the client to release emotions that are stored with the submerged memory or trauma – always a good sign in this kind of regression session.

The release of stored emotions can often have a very cathartic effect. During our therapy sessions, the uncovered trauma was released and processed, and the sleep problem disappeared with it. He was able to sleep through the night from then on without waking.

This case study highlights the need for a one-to-one hypnotherapy session to resolve a sleep problem with a very specific root cause. In this type of case, it is unlikely a hypnosis audio alone will solve the problem, as the underlying root cause isn't being addressed.

Why do we dream?

From the beginning of time, every civilisation has had its theories on dreaming. In many ancient cultures, it was believed that dreaming was the conduit for the gods to relay messages to us about the future. Other ancient cultures believed that the spirit left the body during sleep, enabling it to visit other dimensions such as the astral plane. Sigmund Freud, the grandfather of modern psychology, brought the notion of dreaming back to the forefront of discussion in the late-nineteenth century. He believed that dreams were the route into the deeper depths of the human psyche.

In spite of our amazing advances over the last 100 years, we are still not much further on in understanding why we dream. Some believe that dreaming allows us to house-clean our mind and process information, which we then store in our unconscious mind. Others believe that dreaming allows the higher self to connect to other dimensions so that the spirit is free to travel, or that our dreams are our true suppressed feelings. Some people believe dreams can offer insights into our future, but the truth is, however, no one really knows why we dream.

Controlling our dreams

Lucid dreams are dreams that you can actually step into and control. They are wonderful experiences that seem to occur in lighter sleep states. You are fully aware of what is happening in a lucid dream and also aware of the fact that you are dreaming. In psychology, this is referred to as meta-awareness. Lucid dreams are also usually very vivid and positive in nature, and are often bright, colourful affairs. They frequently relate to events in our lives. It is as though we can resolve problems through these dreams.

The Lucid Dream technique will help to encourage you to actively take control of your dreams and find solutions to problems.

★★★ Animal sleep fact

The species who are champions of sleep are sloths, who spend 80 per cent of their lives asleep. Close behind on 75 per cent are armadillos and some species of bat. At the other end of the chart are animals that get by on just three to four hours a night. These include elephants, horses, donkeys, cows, sheep, goats, deer and giraffes.

Lucid Dream technique

Close your eyes and begin to breathe very slowly and deeply. Allow your mind to become still and quiet, and relax every muscle in your body from the top of your head to the tips of your toes. Take as long as you need to do this and feel all the tension disappear from your body.

Now you can guide yourself into a deeper level of self-hypnosis by silently and mentally counting down from ten to one. Leave about five seconds between each number and feel every muscle in your body relax more and more. Maybe you can imagine yourself going down a beautiful, grand staircase with each descending number. Feel yourself drifting down into deeper and deeper levels of mental and physical relaxation.

Now count down again but this time repeat the affirmations that follow: ten...nine...Say the affirmation 'I feel creative and inspired.' Eight...seven...'I love to dream.' Six...five...'I have so much potential inside.' Four...three...'I can control my dreams when I sleep.' Two...one...Go deeper and deeper to that powerful and resourceful part of you.

At this point, you should be deeply relaxed and in the ideal state to absorb affirmations. I want you to repeat the following affirmations very slowly and with real intent. Say these affirmations with real feeling and emotion. Imagine every part of you repeating the affirmations with complete conviction. Take a slow, deep breath after each affirmation. Repeat this sequence a dozen or more times. The length of time is not important – what is important is that you really feel these words are a reality.

I am in full control of my dreams when I sleep.
I find solutions and answers in my dreams.
I wake up in the morning feeling creative and inspired.
I love to dream.

At this point, you can let your imagination drift so that you can maybe find the answer to a problem without actually thinking about it. Just place your trust in finding solutions or answers in this pleasant, sleepy dream.

When you are ready, you can naturally drift off into a deep sleep where your lucid dreaming may well occur.

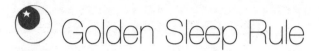 Golden Sleep Rule

2. Sleep in darkness and silence.

When you go to bed, you must sleep in complete darkness so that not even the LED from your alarm can be seen. If you have an alarm with an LED, turn it round so that it cannot be seen at all.

Make sure that you turn off all lights outside your room. Minimise all sound inside and outside your bedroom. Make sure your curtains are thick enough to block out early-morning light, unless of course you plan to rise at sunrise each day.

Chapter 2

WHAT HAPPENS IF WE DON'T GET ENOUGH SLEEP?

Sleep debt

Most people nowadays get insufficient sleep, both in quantity and quality. The evidence of this is that many people experience daytime tiredness, which is completely unnatural. Sleep, along with good diet and exercise, is not given the importance in our lives that it deserves. When you get these three things right, along with a positive mindset and emotional stability, you will be as healthy as you can possibly be.

As mentioned, everyone needs a different amount of sleep each night. For most of us, it is between six and eight hours. If we ever sleep for less than our specific sleep requirement, we start to accumulate what is known as sleep debt. So if you need eight hours of sleep and you only get seven hours, then you have a sleep debt of an hour, which will need to be caught up on in the near future. Sleep debt accumulates, builds quickly and does not decrease of its own accord. The longer a person stays awake, the more sleep they will require to rectify this.

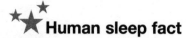

Human sleep fact

Parents of new babies each miss approximately 400–700 hours of sleep in the first year.

However, the old saying 'You can't make up lost sleep' is not true. A seven-day week with Sunday as the day for rest and relaxation is part of our historical heritage. Even the Bible states that God worked for six days and rested on the seventh. There was good logic behind this: we need a day of recuperation to catch up on any sleep debt and recharge our batteries. The Sunday lie-in is a typical example of a way in which we repay our sleep debt – and if this worked for God, you can be sure it will work for us mere mortals!

Another example of catching up on lost sleep is when we are on holiday. When we are not governed by time, we sleep longer. More often than not, though, sleep debt resolves itself naturally as the body will react to a lack of sleep by having daytime drowsiness, creating an intense desire to sleep. This forces us to catnap, go to sleep early or sleep in late. To a degree, using self-hypnosis to still the mind can also help to resolve sleep debt, as when you are in that deeply relaxed state, you allow the mind and body to recharge in much the same way as when you sleep.

☽ Self-Hypnosis ☽
Recharge technique

This technique is ideal if you are feeling tired and you need to recharge. If you are not getting enough sleep and don't have the opportunity to catch up on your sleep debt, use self-hypnosis during the day. If you are working, a lunchtime break is an ideal opportunity to try this. Do it directly after eating your lunch.

After 10 or 20 minutes of being in this calm and centred space, you will feel energised, clearer in your mind and much more effective in your work. You will also go some way towards clearing your sleep debt.

Go to a quiet place, get into a comfortable sitting or preferably lying position and close your eyes. Don't worry if there are distractions nearby; just calm your mind by breathing slowly and deeply in through your nose and out through your mouth. Feel all the muscles in your body relax with each slow out-breath and allow your mind to become still and quiet. Stay in this quiet, still space for 10 minutes or as long as feasible. You can use this or any of the longer self-hypnosis techniques in this book if you have more time.

It has been said that Margaret Thatcher got by on four hours' sleep a night but made up her sleep debt by doing something similar to the above technique for 20 minutes each day. Love her or loathe her, she got a lot done on four hours' kip a night.

Sleep deprivation

Sleep deprivation affects our mental functioning far more than our physical functioning. When we are seriously sleep-deprived, the brain almost switches off, Cognitive functions, concentration and co-ordination become very difficult. In a sleep-deprived state, however, we can still summon extra energy to perform manual tasks. It may explain why mountaineers and people who get lost in remote terrains have the physical stamina to endure all kinds of challenges but suffer mental fatigue and make poor decisions.

When we are sleep-deprived, it becomes impossible to ignore, as our ability to function normally is eroded. This can manifest itself in poor decision-making, impaired judgement, lack of attention to detail and stifling of creativity. At times, people can even look drunk or ill. Studies show that the longer we are sleep-deprived, the stronger the urge to sleep becomes. An

★ ★
★ Human sleep fact

As a group, 18- to 24-year-olds deprived of sleep suffer more from impaired performance than older adults.

example many can relate to is feeling sleepy when driving alone on a long, boring motorway journey. In spite of the obvious danger of falling asleep while driving at high speed, the desire to sleep can feel overwhelming. In these situations, it is wise to pull over and grab some catch-up sleep in a service-station car park.

Sleep deprivation records

There are a number of cases of people who have attempted to stay awake for as long as possible, usually to set records or become famous. In 1959, an American disc jockey called Peter Tripp had his 15 minutes of fame for staying awake under supervision for eight consecutive days and nights. However, he paid a heavy price for this feat of endurance. As the days went on, it became increasingly hard for those around him to keep him awake. After three days, Tripp became abusive and unpleasant, and after five days, his grip on reality became diminished and he suffered from bouts of hallu-cinations, paranoia and delusions. His physiological symptoms included a continuous decline in body temperature, and towards the end of the experiment, his brainwave patterns were virtually indistinguishable from those of a sleeping person, even though he appeared to be awake. After 201 hours, he had broken the existing record. He then fell into a deep sleep, lasting 24 hours. When he awoke, his hallucinations and paranoia had gone, but the experience had a profound effect on his life. His friends and family felt he was a changed man and not for the better. His wife left him, he lost his job as a disc jockey, and he became a drifter. The moral of this story is don't intentionally attempt long-term sleep deprivation if you are married and have a job that you like!

As with all endurance tests, there is always someone who will want to take it one step further. In 1965, a 17-year-old high-school student called Randy Gardner got himself into the record books for lasting a monumental 11 days and nights without sleep. Scientists from Stanford University closely monitored his 264-hour sleep-deprivation marathon. Once again his lack of sleep had adverse side-effects, including blurred vision, irritability, slurred speech, memory lapses and hallucinations. At one point, he believed he was a famous footballer. However, unlike Tripp, he suffered no long-term consequences and recovered fully.

These experiments serve to highlight the fact that sleep deprivation is very debilitating and can cause all kinds of problems. It has even been used as a form of torture. In China, it was used on prisoners awaiting capital punishment, so that they would suffer maximum torment before death. Some of the more unsavoury police interrogators in certain countries still use sleep deprivation to get information from prisoners. Systematic sleep deprivation is said to be one of the most effective forms of coercion. When people are woken suddenly and randomly at odd hours over a period of time, they begin to lose their normal, rational faculties and become very vulnerable. Even the strongest people become weak and debilitated under this kind of pressure, as their ability to reason and think logically rapidly diminishes. In these circumstances, sleep deprivation leaves people without the ability to make sound judgements. In a sense, they lose their grip on reality. By losing track of time and with an internal body clock in turmoil, sleep-deprived prisoners become much easier to interrogate and manipulate, and to be forced into making admissions.

This must be the same reason my son asks me to lend him money when I'm tired. I always knew he was a smart kid.

Sleep deprivation and accidents

Sleeplessness is also a major cause of accidents and injuries. The 1989 *Exxon Valdez* oil spill off the coast of Alaska, the *Challenger* space shuttle disaster and the Chernobyl nuclear accident have all been attributed to human errors in which sleep-deprivation played a role. It is a fact that tiredness is responsible for far more road accidents than alcohol or drugs. In Canada, a study showed that the extra hour of sleep received when clocks are put back at the start of daylight was found to coincide with a fall in the number of road accidents.

In 2001, a sleep-deprived driver fell asleep at the wheel and crashed into a railway line, causing a catastrophic train crash near Selby that killed ten people. The driver admitted that he had had no sleep the night before, but claimed he could still drive safely. He received a prison sentence for what was an accident, but it was made worse by his assertion that his extreme lack of sleep was not a major factor in causing the accident.

Sleep deprivation has strong similarities with the state of being inebriated. As well as impairing performance and clouding our judgement, it fuels recklessness and, for reasons unknown, can fire up libidinous desires. And it can hamper our ability to realise that our senses are not as sharp as they should be. All of these characteristics are common in both drunkenness and sleep deprivation, and both states lead to a feeling of being hungover.

Microsleeps

Microsleeps occur when people become overtired. They are brief episodes of drowsiness and loss of attention that manifest in behaviours such as the blank stare, head snapping and spontaneous eye closure. This can occur when a person is fatigued but trying to stay awake to perform a monotonous task like driving a car or watching TV.

Microsleeps can last for a few seconds or for several minutes, and often the person is not aware that they have drifted off to sleep. They can even occur when a person's eyes are open – similar to a daydreaming or hypnosis state. The physical manifestation of a microsleep is when people fail to respond to outside information like traffic lights changing or a phone ringing.

★ Human sleep fact

It is estimated that sleep deprivation accounts for one in six fatal road accidents.

Although microsleeps are a result of being sleep-deprived or in sleep debt, they are more likely to happen at certain times of the day, such as the pre-dawn and mid-afternoon hours, when our body temperature is lower and our circadian rhythm is in a dip. Microsleeps increase with cumulative sleep debt. In other words, the more sleep-deprived a person is, the greater the chance a microsleep episode will occur.

Beauty sleep

For those of us who won't see 30 again, the effects of poor sleep can be seen in the physical form of bags under the eyes, pronounced lines and wrinkles. When sleep problems occur over a long period of time, it can rapidly speed up the ageing process. The parallels between sleeplessness and ageing are in part because the effects of both impair the pre-frontal cortex – the region of your brain that is very active when you are awake.

Lack of sleep has also been shown to cause skin disorders in both animals and humans. Another less obvious problem that is in part aggravated by sleep deprivation is the onset of breasts and pot-bellies in middle-aged men. This is because men produce their growth hormone almost exclusively when they sleep. When a man is sleep-deprived therefore, his body will not be producing enough of the growth hormone. Scientists believe that this is a factor in turning muscle into flab. For men to avoid blobbing out in middle age, good sleep is a must.

Sleeping for less than your personal requirement over prolonged periods will undoubtedly detract from your looks. Unfortunately, sleeping for hours on end will not enhance your physical attributes, which is a pity! For advice on how to calculate how much sleep you need, see page 171.

The beauty sleep supercharge

If you have a big celebration or a wedding coming up, you will want to be at your best, so a good night's sleep is vital. Follow these steps on the day before any big event:

- Do not drink any tea, coffee or alcohol, and avoid sugar and salt.

- Have a light meal early in the evening. Avoid meat or anything hard to digest.

- Drink lots of water during the morning and afternoon.

- Exercise during the day as much as possible. In the evening, wind down with some gentle exercise, like yoga.

- Avoid watching TV and minimise computer use, certainly in the evening.

- Before bed, have a warm bath with lavender oil. Add a sprinkle of lavender to your pillow.

- Go to bed early.

- When you get into bed, run through the following day's events in your mind and visualise everything in a very positive light. See yourself on top form and feeling really good in yourself. Use all of your senses to make this real. You may want to use the Future Event Visualisation technique on page 125.

- Don't think about the following day too much, other than when you use the above technique. Thinking about it on a conscious level can create unwanted pressure, whereas visualising the day in a 20-minute self-hypnosis session will set you up to be at your very best.

If after your visualisation you still need help getting to sleep, listen to the *Sleep Well* audio session.

Sleep, health and longevity

Sleep is one of the main cornerstones of our health. It has been shown that longevity goes hand in hand with healthy living, and the main factors are healthy eating, regular exercise, a positive mindset and healthy sleep patterns. If you get those four right, you will probably never know the name of your doctor.

Studies have shown that people who live longer tend to go to sleep earlier and generally have good sleeping patterns.

Some studies have shown that insufficient sleep is linked to increased risk of weight gain, depression, colon cancer, breast cancer, heart disease, stroke and diabetes, so you can see how important it is that you get it right, especially when you consider that these diseases are on the increase.

Excessive sleeping

Regularly sleeping for too long is as bad for our health as sleeping too little. One specific study found that when people sleep less than four hours or, at the other end of the scale, more than ten hours a night, there is a higher than average risk of dying prematurely. In another study of elderly British people, it was found that those who spent 12 hours or more a day in bed had a significantly higher mortality rate than those who spent the average eight hours. Experiments have shown that when people sleep for too long, it can also have a detrimental effect on their health.

If you have the odd day where you sleep for ten hours, it is more than likely you are repaying your sleep debt. It would only be a problem if this lengthy sleeping pattern continued for a long period.

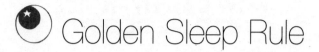 Golden Sleep Rule

3. Avoid consuming food or drink before bedtime.

Do not eat or drink anything other than water for at least four hours before you go to bed at night. For example, if you go to bed at 11 p.m., finish your evening meal by 7 p.m. and avoid anything heavy that takes the body a long time to digest.

Chapter 3

HOW CAN HYPNOSIS HELP ME SLEEP?

What is hypnosis?

The *Sleep Well* audio download that accompanies this book will guide you into a deep state of hypnosis, and many of the self-hypnosis techniques in this book will take you into an altered state of consciousness. The following few pages provide some information on hypnosis and how it is particularly effective in freeing you from poor sleep habits and helping to create good-quality sleep patterns.

Hypnosis is an altered state of consciousness during which suggestions are given to the subject. Suggestions can be given and acted on in normal waking consciousness, but they are far more effective when delivered to a person in an altered state brought on by a hypnotic induction.

The majority of you will only have to listen to the *Sleep Well* recording that comes with this book to know that hypnosis exists. For those of you still unconvinced, consider these often quoted words 'For those who believe, no explanation is necessary; for those who do not believe, no explanation will suffice.'

People sometimes shy away from hypnosis; often this is because they misunderstand what it actually is. Hypnosis stage shows in which hypnotists entertain by using members of the audience who are most susceptible to their suggestions often create a misconception about hypnosis. In these shows, it often appears as though the hypnotist has *all* the power. Many stage hypnotists will actively cultivate a powerful image, but in reality this is an illusion. There is a degree of control and manipulation in this type of show, but it is not always as it seems. Firstly, the vast majority of any audience will not make good subjects for hypnotic stage shows, as not everyone is up for making pillocks of themselves in front of a large audience, so the stage hypnotist will do a number of tests on the audience to find the people who are most likely to follow their every suggestion. These suggestions often get more outrageous as the show progresses, and the hypnotist will hone in on the subjects who have previously followed their suggestions most readily. Stage hypnotists often call these people the stars of the show. They are generally keen to be part of the performance from the beginning and will become more and more compelled to follow the increasingly absurd suggestions given by the stage hypnotist.

I'm not against hypnosis being used for enter-tainment as long as it is used carefully and all sugges-tions are removed at the end of the show. On the positive side, stage hypnosis does highlight the power of deliv-ering hypnotic suggestion and gives people a greater awareness of hypnosis in general. On the downside, people often confuse stage hypnosis with the problem-solving hypnotherapy that I use: I have spent way too much time reassuring people that I won't make them dance around like a chicken! The distinction between stage hypnosis and hypnotherapy is that the former uses hypnosis to entertain, while the latter uses it to help and heal.

The misunderstanding of hypnosis also comes from the way that it is portrayed in the media. Stories about hypnosis only tend to make the news if there has been a problem or it has been misused. If hypnosis features in TV programmes, it is often portrayed with a dramatic twist. In reality, it works very simply. In a professional one-to-one situation, hypnosis is achieved by using various techniques to guide the client into deeper levels of relaxation. It is often a gentle progression from waking consciousness to a deep level of relaxation, rather than a flashy click of the fingers.

When you are in a hypnotic state, you will still be

aware of your surroundings even as you drift into deeper states. It can sometimes feel as though very little is happening and that you can open your eyes at any time and be wide awake. This is because being in hypnosis doesn't feel unusual. It doesn't create a special feeling and so people often don't realise when they are under hypnosis.

When you are in a deep level of mental and physical relaxation, you become receptive to suggestions. Accepting suggestions is the key to using hypnosis as a therapeutic tool. A post-hypnotic suggestion is one that will be acted upon at a later time. For example, a post-hypnotic suggestion could be 'As soon as your head touches the pillow each night, you will find it easy to go into a deep, relaxing sleep.' When a suggestion like this is accepted by your unconscious mind, the next time you go to bed and your head touches the pillow, you will indeed find it easy to go to sleep.

⟩ Elevator Visualisation ⟩
technique

This technique will help you when you are lying in bed at night and your mind is busy.

Close your eyes and begin breathing slowly and deeply in through your nose and out through your mouth. Breathe away any tension with every out-breath. Do this for about ten minutes, then imagine getting into a large, luxurious elevator that goes down ten floors. With each number down from ten to one you drift further towards sleep. When you reach the number one, you will feel very sleepy. The elevator then opens and in front of you is a huge, comfortable bed, which you lazily climb into and go into a deep, deep sleep.

Visualise this clearly and put your feelings into it. Use all of your senses to strengthen the visualisation. For example, notice the smell of the elevator and the warmth of the bed. As you create the pictures in your mind, you will feel very sleepy.

When you visualise, your mind doesn't distinguish between what is real and what is imagined, so when you create visualisations like this, your mind and body will respond positively.

Using hypnosis to create healthy sleep patterns

Using hypnosis to help people overcome problems can be very successful, and it is completely safe when administered by a well-qualified and experienced hypnotherapist. In my hypnotherapy practice, sleep disorders are some of the most common problems I help people with, as hypnotherapy is an extremely effective way of helping people into regular healthy sleep patterns.

Being in an altered state of consciousness, or in a hypnotic trance, is actually something you will experience naturally many times in your life. For example, just before you fall asleep each night and before you are fully awake in the morning, you are in a trance state. Everyone on the planet experiences this. These morning and evening trance states are called the hypnogogic and hypnopompic states. Daydreaming is another naturally occurring trance state that is familiar to all of us. Now you can learn how to create those states at will to empower yourself and develop healthy new sleep patterns.

When you go to sleep at night and you drift from consciousness to unconsciousness, it feels natural, but as you drift off to sleep, your brainwaves are actually slowing. When you go into a hypnotic trance, exactly the same thing happens. So the reason hypnosis is so effective in helping people to sleep well is because it has the same effect on brainwave cycles as when a person goes to sleep naturally.

To give you a clearer idea of the similarity between hypnosis and sleep, let us look in more detail at the brain cycle. The brain cycle states that define our levels of consciousness are referred to as the beta, alpha, theta and delta states. Think of, or visualise, the word 'batted' and you will always remember the sequence of these four states.

When we go to bed and wind down before going to sleep, we are likely to be in a low beta state. When we close our eyes and relax, our brainwaves will descend from beta through alpha and theta to delta when we fall asleep. The ideal state for absorbing visualisations, suggestions and affirmations is between the alpha and theta states. This means that you, me and the Queen experience naturally occurring hypnotic trance states every day. Remember, each and every one of us experiences these four states of consciousness every night when we sleep, so hypnosis simply simulates being asleep, which is why it is so helpful to solving sleep problems.

- The **beta** state is when we are awake and fully conscious. Our brainwaves range from 15 to 40 cycles per second. If we are very alert or engaged in a stimulating mental or physical activity, our brainwaves will be at the higher end of this range.

- The **alpha** state has a frequency range from 9 to 14 cycles per second. This is where a person is mentally relaxed or in a state of light meditation. You are still aware of everything around you, but your mind is calm and you feel physically relaxed. Daydreaming is typical of the alpha state, and you are also more receptive to hypnotic suggestions and affirmations in this state.

- **Theta** brainwaves are typically between five and eight cycles per second. This is the state you achieve when you are in deeper hypnosis or close to falling asleep. In this very relaxed theta state, hypnotic suggestion can also be given and readily accepted, then acted upon at a later date.

- **Delta** is the final brainwave state with a range of one and a half to four cycles per second. Sleep occurs when our brainwaves slow down to two to three cycles per second. The deepest hypnotic trance state is called somnambulism, which occurs when you are in or close to the delta state.

Chapter 4

COMMON SLEEP PROBLEMS

As we saw in the Introduction, the current predilection for staying awake after dark is a very recent thing. It is only since the advent of electricity that we have taken to staying up late. It has been shown that regular exposure to electric lighting late into the night can alter our internal biological rhythms. Natural daylight resets our biological clock every day, but misleading light cues confuse our circadian rhythms and cause problems like insomnia. In fact, most of our sleep disorders are very modern problems caused by our lifestyles.

Electric lighting has also both directly and indirectly been the cause of many of our modern-day eyesight problems. Eyesight problems often occur because we strain to view things in artificial light and because we spend too long looking at computer and TV screens. Nowadays it is common to see people wearing glasses because of poor eyesight and it is something we have come to accept as normal. But in times gone by, our

Sleeping tablets case study

I recently received a letter from a lady in her seventies who had been on sleeping tablets for 35 years. The lady had started using my Sleep Well programme and was now able to sleep well without the need for tablets. Listening to the audio each night became a natural replacement for her medication. Anyone on sedatives or any long-term medication for sleep should look at alternative solutions. The simple switch from sleeping tablets to using my hypnotherapy recording was the solution in this case.

eyesight was generally much better and we were able to see very well in darkness before the advent of electricity made this unnecessary.

Insomnia

'Insomnia' is the Latin word for sleeplessness. It is a sleep disorder that literally means an inability to sleep or the inability to remain asleep for the correct amount of time needed for your mind and body to rejuvenate.

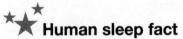

Human sleep fact

Having regular disturbed
or disrupted sleep during
childhood will often lead to the
development of insomnia later
in life.

There are three different types
of insomnia: transient, acute and
chronic. Most people occasionally
suffer from transient insomnia,
due to such causes as jet lag or
short-term anxiety. Transient
insomnia typically lasts from
a single night to a few weeks.
Acute insomnia can last between three weeks to six
months, and the more serious chronic insomnia occurs
nightly for at least a month.

The US Department of Health and Human Services
claims that 20 per cent of people suffer from insomnia
each year, which tends to increase with age and affects
about 40 per cent of women and 30 per cent of men.
Causes of insomnia include fear, depression, physical
pain and an overactive mind. One of the most common
causes is mental tension brought on by anxiety, worries,
overwork, stress and overexcitement. Suppressed
feelings of resentment, anger and bitterness may also
cause insomnia. Physical problems such as constipation,
dyspepsia and habits like overeating at night, excessive
intake of tea or coffee, smoking and going to bed hungry
are among the other causes.

Treating insomnia

Insomnia is a symptom of a problem and not a disease, which in most cases means you can make lifestyle changes that correct the problem. It is nice to know that it is within your control to rectify this problem.

Getting regular healthy sleep is crucial, but sadly, doctors receive very little training in sleep disorders. It is far easier to prescribe drugs that treat the symptoms than to delve deeper and find the root cause.

Chemically produced sedative drugs have the potential of causing psychological dependence – that is to say, the individual cannot accept that they can sleep without drugs. Long-term use of chemical sedatives for sleeping problems can cause imbalances in the body and other unwanted side-effects. If the user is not weaned off the drug in the correct way, they can also suffer withdrawal symptoms.

Many insomniacs rely on sleeping tablets and other sedatives to get rest. The most commonly prescribed drugs for insomnia are the benzodiazepines. This includes drugs such as temazepam, diazepam, lorazepam, flurazepam, nitrazepam and midazolam. These medications can be addictive, especially after taking them over long periods of time. Some sleeping tablets, such as barbiturates, even suppress the all-important REM sleep.

There is so much widespread over-prescribing of drugs that natural options are rarely considered by health professionals. If you are wondering why drugs are over-prescribed and often the only solution offered by doctors and pharmacies, it is because they are big business and medical practitioners and pharmacies are their main outlet. Powerful drug companies rely on huge incomes from sleeping tablets and sedatives. This is all about money. It isn't possible to patent natural alternative remedies for insomnia, which often offer a much safer way to help sleeping problems.

For tens of thousands of years, we have treated illness with diet, natural herbs and minerals, but since the

NOTE: At the time of writing a raft of EU legislation is heading our way that looks set to take control of the alternative natural medicine market. The impact of this new legislation could mean that hundreds of natural vitamin and mineral supplements and common herbal remedies will be banned outright. If these insidious plans succeed, things like vitamin C, ginseng, echinacea and St John's wort will disappear from our health shops. The National Association of Health Food Stores claims that as many as three-quarters of its members could go out of business. The drug companies would then have the market to themselves.

onset of modern medicine, the primary way of treating imbalances and sickness is with chemical drugs. All chemical drugs ever do is treat the symptom of the problem, but to overcome any illness, disease or imbalance in the body, you have to treat the root cause.

Alcohol has sedative properties and can help with the onset of sleep, but it will affect the quality and the depth of sleep. The REM-sleep-suppressing effects of alcohol prevent restful, quality sleep and it is unlikely to lead to dreaming. This is why we often go to sleep easily after consuming alcohol but wake in the middle of the night. The other downsides to using alcohol to sleep are dependency, hangovers and the feeling of grogginess in the morning.

Cannabis oil is now known to act as an effective sleep aid, but smoking marijuana regularly can have complications long term and can lead to psychological dependence, depression, apathy and paranoia.

If you want to get to the bottom of insomnia and cure it, rather than suppressing or controlling the symptoms, then a natural, holistic approach is the only solution. My personal Sleep Well Programme will get you well on the way to creating healthy new sleep patterns.

Sleepwalking

Sleepwalking is a sleep disorder that is characterised by walking, talking and other normal waking activities while the person is asleep or in a sleep-like state. A sleepwalking episode can last just a minute or two, or, in more severe cases, for more than 30 minutes.

Sleepwalking most often occurs during deep non-REM sleep early in the night, but it can also occur during REM sleep near morning. As we saw in Chapter 1: What is Sleep?, normally in these deeper stages of sleep, the brain releases chemicals that send signals to the muscles to remain immobile, mainly so that dreams will not be acted out. However, people who sleepwalk do not have this chemical trigger, which results in them sleepwalking.

Sleepwalkers are not conscious of their actions and rarely recall their sleepwalking episodes. This is why sleepwalking often goes undetected and is only discovered when the sleepwalker is woken or aroused by someone else. Sleepwalking is more commonly experienced in people with high levels of stress, anxiety or psychological factors. Alcohol abuse, brain seizures, drugs and medications can also play a role, as well as genetic factors.

Sleepwalking activity may include a person simply

sitting up in bed or getting up and walking around, or even more complex activities such as going to the bathroom, dressing and undressing. They will appear to be awake, but are actually asleep. It has even been known for people to safely drive a car while sleep-walking. In these cases, their unconscious mind takes over and their ideo-motor responses can control the car without conscious thought. All experienced drivers drive this way when they are awake. Driving a familiar route without conscious analysis is a typical waking trance state that most adults experience.

A common misconception is that sleepwalking is an individual acting out the physical movements within a dream and should not be woken. However, the activity of sleepwalking is not always as a result of responding to dreams and it is not dangerous to wake a sleepwalker. When a sleepwalker is awoken suddenly, it is common for them to be confused or disoriented for a short time.

Tips to help sleepwalking problems

- Being overtired can trigger sleepwalking, so make sure you catch up on your sleep debt by getting plenty of rest. If a sleepwalking habit starts suddenly, maybe consider taking a holiday on which you can get plenty of uninterrupted rest and relaxation.

- If you are a sleepwalker, your bedroom should be on the ground floor of the house as this minimises the danger of falling from open windows. If it is an ongoing severe problem, lock the doors and windows, cover glass windows with heavy drapes and you can even place an alarm or bell on the bedroom door.

- Remove anything from the bedroom that could be dangerous or harmful during a sleepwalking episode.

- Seek out an experienced hypnotherapist who will be able to help get to the root cause of the sleepwalking problem. One-to-one hypnotherapy sessions can be very effective in overcoming sleepwalking disorders in both adults and children. The suggestion 'You will wake fully at the onset of sleepwalking' is very effective under hypnosis. To find a hypnotherapist in the UK, see Further Resources on page 177.

- Review any current drugs or medication. Do your own research and check out any side-effects.

- Avoid any kind of stimuli (auditory or visual) prior to bedtime.

- Develop a calming ritual at bedtime. Any of the tips and general self-hypnosis techniques in this book will help you here, as will the *Sleep Well* audio download.

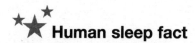 **Human sleep fact**

Older people have more sleep disorders. One reason is because the blood-flow mechanism that transfers body heat to the skin shrinks with age.

Hypnosis and sleepwalking

Being under hypnosis and sleepwalking are very similar states, the main difference being that you are consciously aware of what's happening when you are in a trance state under hypnosis, whereas sleepwalkers typically have no conscious awareness of their state either during or after sleepwalking. The deepest hypnosis state and sleepwalking are trance states that are both referred to as somnambulism, and this is where the brain is in the delta state of one and a half to four brainwave cycles per second. For more information on the different sleep states, see page 58.

☽ Self-hypnosis Sleepwalking ☽ technique

Use any of the previous mental and physical relaxation techniques beginning with slow, deep, circular breathing. You don't need to become too deeply relaxed; just get into a pleasant state of relaxation so that you feel calm and centred. Now still your mind for a few moments and repeat the following affirmations over and over in a slow, steady mantra. As always, put your feelings into the affirmations as you repeat them, as this makes them strong and anchors them deeply in your unconscious mind.

I sleep safely every night.

I always wake up immediately if I sleepwalk.

After affirming to yourself, you can let go and drift off to sleep with the knowledge that your unconscious mind will wake you if you sleepwalk.

Sleep apnea

This is a condition that occurs when breathing is interrupted during sleep, which then interrupts the normal sleep cycle. There are three types of sleep apnea: obstructive, central and mixed. Each type has a different root cause. Obstructive sleep apnea is caused by the air being unable to flow to the lungs from the mouth or nose due to physical obstruction or lack of effort. People with obstructive sleep apnea are often not aware of this occurrence, but they complain of excessive sleepiness during the day. In central sleep apnea, the airway is not blocked, but the brain fails to send the signal for the muscles to breathe, causing pauses in breath. Central sleep apnea interrupts the normal breathing stimulus of the central nervous system, and the individual must actually wake up to resume breathing. Mixed apnea, as the name implies, is a combination of the two.

Hereditary or genetic physical attributes can play a part in sleep apnea, such as a relatively small airway between the mouth and throat area. Naturally large tonsils or adenoids may also cause disruption in air flow to the lungs, causing pauses in breath.

Symptoms of sleep apnea can include loud snoring, dry or parched throat on waking, gasping for breath or choking, poor quality of sleep, memory problems, morning headaches, irritation, impaired concentration, depression and mood swings.

With each type of apnoea, people stop breathing repeatedly during their sleep, sometimes hundreds of times during the night and often for a minute or longer. When this happens, the brain briefly arouses the person in order for them to resume breathing. This is the brain's unconscious survival mechanism working perfectly, but consequently, sufferers of sleep apnea often have fragmented, poor-quality sleep.

You are more at risk of sleep apnoea if you are overweight, male and over the age of forty, although sleep apnea can strike anyone at any age, even children. Untreated, sleep apnoea can cause high blood pressure, heart attacks, strokes, memory problems, weight gain, premature ageing, impotency and headaches.

Remedies for sleep apnea include losing weight, eliminating tobacco, alcohol and sleeping pills. If you do suffer with sleep apnea, try to change sleeping positions to ensure regular breathing and avoid sleeping on your back. To help this, you can place a small ball in a sock and tie it across your waist so the ball rests on your back.

> **The lion and the calf shall lie down together, but the calf won't get much sleep.**
>
> *Woody Allen*

Fear of the dark case study

Sleep problems can stem from a wide variety of causes. One of the most unusual client sessions I have experienced was with a lady who came to see me because she had a fear of the dark. She explained that as soon as it became dark each night, she would feel anxious and sometimes have panic attacks if she was home alone. As you can imagine, a fear of the dark is very debilitating because night-time is obviously unavoidable.

This lady had tried other therapies and medical help without success and had turned to hypnotherapy as a last resort. With most types of fear hypnotherapy works well in getting to the root cause and making changes at a core level. Almost all fears and phobias are learned and under hypnosis they can be unlearned and replaced with a new positive pattern of behaviour.

I followed a well-proven technique to regress her to the cause of the problem. When she was in a deeply relaxed state, I gave her the key suggestion – 'When I count to three, you will go back to the first time you experienced a fear of the dark.' With that, she regressed back to a time in her past when the problem began. I won't go into detail here regarding this session, as it was a very personal experience, but I was able to guide her to let go of any negative feelings and emotions connected to her past experience. I then gave her suggestions that she would now be free of her fear. At the right time, I guided her back to full waking consciousness.

When the lady returned for a second session a week later, she told me that for the first time in years she was now able to sleep through the night without any fear. That first session had been entirely successful and the fear had disappeared.

The root causes of fears and anxieties are often unique to a person's past experiences, so solutions I find to people's problems are generally very different. You cannot underestimate the effectiveness of hypnotherapy in overcoming fears and problem patterns of behaviour. As babies, we are born perfect and it is only experience that teaches us fear and anxiety. Even so, whatever fears we learn can be unlearned. Hypnotherapy is at its most effective when changing destructive behavioural patterns and replacing them with positive solutions.

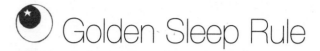 Golden Sleep Rule

4. Write a to-do list.

Keep a notepad and pen by your bedside so that you can jot down things you need to do the next day. Once you have written them on your pad, you can forget about them and go to sleep safe in the knowledge that what you have written down will be remembered. A to-do list will help you switch off from any worries and go to sleep feeling more organised.

If you tend to mull over problems or get unwanted thoughts at night, then you must also use the Clearing Your Mind technique on page 132.

SECTION 2

THE SLEEP WELL
PROGRAMME

Chapter 5

GETTING STARTED

The Sleep Well Programme contains everything you need to cure your problem. It is split into six steps: practical remedies, the ultimate hydration remedy, the ultimate healthy-eating remedy, the ultimate exercise remedy, the ultimate natural remedies and the ultimate self-hypnosis remedy.

Before you get started on curing your sleep difficulties, however, it is vital that you establish what the problem areas are for you. For this reason, I have devised a checklist to help you identify the root causes of your issues.

Checklist of the causes of sleep problems

Below is a list of things that can cause sleep problems. Take a good look at the different areas and score each one between one and ten.

Diet

If you completely avoid all junk food, sugar, salt, tea, coffee, alcohol, fizzy drinks and only drink fresh mineral water and eat raw, organic, healthy food in small amounts, then you can score ten. (That will just be Gillian McKeith, then!) If you consume most types of junk food and drinks in a typical week, your score will be one. Think about your diet over a typical week and make an honest assessment, where ten is as healthy as it gets and one is very unhealthy.

| 1 | 2 | 3 | 4 | 5 | 6 | 7 | 8 | 9 | 10 |
| □ | □ | □ | □ | □ | □ | □ | □ | □ | □ |

Exercise

If you leap out of bed early each morning and begin a long exercise workout, then exercise again in the afternoon and evening, you can score ten. (That will just be overly sincere Americans on shopping channels who sell exercise gismos!) Typically, if you exercise four or five times a week and this includes a mixture of activities, like yoga, swimming, cycling and jogging, your score will be around seven or eight. If you do no exercise, drive everywhere and slob out in front of the TV every night, your score will be one. Think about how much you exercise in a typical week and score accordingly.

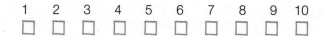

Electromagnetic fields (EMFs)

If you have no TVs, phones, radios or any electrical devices in your bedroom, including electric alarm clocks, then you can score ten. If you have all of these things, your score will be one. Check now how many electrical devices you have in your bedroom and score accordingly.

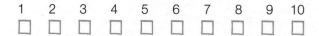

Environmental

If you live in an area with no noise pollution or light pollution, you can score ten. This would typically be a cottage in the countryside surrounded by fields. If you live next to a main road in a busy town centre with lots of noise and traffic pollution, your score will be one.

Mark your score depending on how healthy your environment is.

1   2   3   4   5   6   7   8   9   10
☐   ☐   ☐   ☐   ☐   ☐   ☐   ☐   ☐   ☐

Lifestyle

If you are very happy in your work and home life, and your relationships with everyone around you are perfect, then score ten. If your personal relationships are all in a mess, you hate your work and drown your sorrows in alcohol or smoke Jamaican woodbines for escapism each night, your score will be one. Mark your score depending on how healthy your lifestyle is.

1   2   3   4   5   6   7   8   9   10
☐   ☐   ☐   ☐   ☐   ☐   ☐   ☐   ☐   ☐

Stress

If you love life, are eternally optimistic and positive, and can easily cope with pressure, then score ten. If you are a deeply pessimistic person who struggles to cope with pressure and feels constantly stressed, your score will be one.

1   2   3   4   5   6   7   8   9   10
☐   ☐   ☐   ☐   ☐   ☐   ☐   ☐   ☐   ☐

Busy mind

If you are laid-back and never have a care in the world, then score ten. If you constantly worry, mull over situations late at night and can never make decisions because your mind is always full, your score will be one.

1   2   3   4   5   6   7   8   9   10
☐   ☐   ☐   ☐   ☐   ☐   ☐   ☐   ☐   ☐

Now total up your score.

If you scored above 50 and are having sleep problems, it may be that there are unresolved issues from your past hampering your sleep patterns. In this case, you will need to delve deeper to find the root cause of your problems. As seen in the case study about the unconscious mind on page 31, one-to-one hypnotherapy can work well in uncovering the cause of problems that may be out of your conscious awareness. There is always a reason behind every problem, and you need to get to the bottom of it. See Further Resources on page 174, where you will find advice on locating a well-qualified hypnotherapist who can help you.

If you scored between 35 and 50, you will fall into the category where there is room for improvement. Maybe there is no underlying single root cause of your sleep problems – it could just be a cumulative effect. Look at the areas on the checklist where your score was five or less and use the Sleep Well Programme to work on remedying the problems in these individual areas.

If you scored less than 35, you need help now! Look at the areas where you scored poorly and make changes. You have to do this if you want to give yourself the opportunity to sleep well at night. It is easy to make lifestyle changes. You simply **make a decision to do it** and then use a little determination to remain on course.

The six steps in the Sleep Well Programme, covered over the following pages, will help you. I have also produced many hypnosis recordings covering everything from weight loss to exercise motivation. These hypnosis audios can help you in specific areas for reinforcing your determination to make changes. See Further Resources on page 175, where I have listed some additional reading, audios, DVDs and apps that may be of use.

Chapter 6

THE SLEEP WELL PROGRAMME – STEP 1

Step 1: Practical remedies to cure sleep problems

Now you have completed the checklist in the previous chapter, you should have a much clearer idea of where your specific problems lie. In the first step of my unique Sleep Well Programme, we will address these key problem areas. Pay most attention to any area where your checklist score was low. If it means redecorating your bedroom or buying new thick curtains, then you must do this as each one of these small steps is going to add up to a lasting holistic solution.

Diet and exercise

For practical advice on diet and exercise, see Chapter 7: Steps 2, 3 and 4 of the Sleep Well Programme.

Electromagnetic fields (EMFs)

1 **Remove anything that emits EMFs**. Make sure your bedroom is free of all electrical equipment, such as TVs, DVDs, stereos and computers and anything that emits electromagnetic energy. Remove mobile or cordless phones from anywhere near your bedside when you sleep. The only exception to this would be an electric lamp, but try and use one that has soft lighting. If it seems a wrench to remove your plasma from your bedroom wall, just think how important your sleep is. You need to prioritise and give yourself every chance of getting into a regular healthy sleep routine, which will help you be so much more productive in your daily life. For more information, see 'What effect do electromagnetic fields have on sleep?' in Chapter 10.

2 **Buy a natural daylight alarm clock**, which slowly turns off the light at night and on in the morning, giving a similar effect to sunrise and sunset. They can be a little expensive, but you can't put too high a price on sleeping well. They are also much more conducive to natural sleep patterns than an alarm clock or clock radio. To learn more about daylight alarm clocks, see the box on page 139.

Environmental

1 **Sleep in absolute darkness**. There must be no light from
other rooms. Light affects our circadian rhythms, which affect
our body temperature, organ function and ability to sleep.
Even very small rays of light from a digital alarm clock can
be enough to disrupt the sleep cycle. The dim light turns off
a neural switch in the brain, causing levels of a key sleep
chemical to rapidly decline. You may well remain asleep
through this, but your sleep cycles are being hampered. If
your alarm clock has an LED, you must turn it away so that it
is out of your direct eyesight. Studies have shown that even
LEDs can interfere with sleep. Make sure you are not close to
any light, no matter how dim or innocuous it may seem. Your
curtains must also be thick enough to block out any light.
Complete darkness will undoubtedly help to improve the
quality of your sleep.

2 **Ensure your bed is comfortable.** If your bed is worn out or
uncomfortable, then it is not going to help you sleep well.
When you do need to buy a new bed, it is worth remembering
that you are going to spend a third of your life in it – or over
twenty-five years! – so don't skimp on it: buy the very best bed
that you can afford. In an age where many get financed up to
the hilt to buy fancy cars or plasma TVs, essentials like a good-
quality bed should be at the top of any financial planning.

3 **Invest in good-quality pillows and sheets.** Research shows that synthetic pillows house more bacteria and dust mites than good-quality feather pillows. You will also keep the mites at bay if you use very high-quality sheets made from finely woven materials. Luxury sheets and feather pillows will also feel more comfortable against your skin and so help you sleep.

4 **Turn your mattress over every six months.** You can get more life out of your bed this way, and it will stop your mattress becoming lumpy, which can hinder sleep.

5 **Make sure your pillows and mattress are clean.** Change your sheets and pillowcases regularly.

6 **Reduce air pollution.** If you live in an environment that is polluted, buy an air-purifying device for your bedroom.

7 **Create the ideal bedroom for sleep.** Your bedroom's colours and general décor should be conducive to relaxation and sleep. Decorate in soft colours, such as green, blue, pink, white or lilac. Green and blue are ideal. Green reflects nature and has soothing properties that promote balance, harmony and peace. Blue gives a vibe of space, coolness, well-being and serenity. Colours that have a stimulating effect, like bright reds, oranges or yellows, must be avoided.

8 **Make sure you are not too warm or too cold in bed.**
   Maintaining a good temperature in bed will help you sleep.
   Don't have too many covers or a duvet that is too warm, but
   also make sure your covers don't leave you feeling slightly
   cold.

9 **Minimise noise.** Make sure your bedroom is as quiet as
   possible. Thick curtains are a must if you live in an area
   with a lot of noise or near a busy road. To eliminate all
   noise, consider using earplugs. They can also help if your
   partner snores. Use a comfortable light-blocking sleep mask
   to eliminate light. This is useful if your partner comes to bed
   at a later time than you. Studies have found that exposure
   to noise at night can suppress immune function even if the
   sleeper doesn't wake up.

★★★ Human sleep fact

Unfamiliar noise during the first and last two hours of sleep has
the greatest disruptive effect on the sleep cycle.

Lifestyle and stress

1 **Relax before bedtime.** Avoid watching TV in the evening for
two nights a week or as often as you can. Instead, read a book
or spend a relaxing evening doing things that won't stimulate
your mind. Even if you can do this once or twice a week, it is
highly likely that you will sleep well on the nights when your
mind is not bombarded with TV imagery. Try it and see how
different it feels.

2 **Avoid stress** as much as possible by listening to relaxation
audios, exercising, having fun, eating healthily, meditating,
playing sport, practising yoga, tai chi or any relaxation
exercise. If stress is a particular problem for you, look at the
advice in Chapter 9: Overcoming the Worries that Keep Us
Awake, which will help you to deal with the common worries
that cause sleepless nights.

3 **Revere your sleep.** It is so important for you to get a full
night's sleep. Make sure that this is a priority in your life. If
ever you have a sleep-deprived night, make plans to redeem
this the next night so that you are never in sleep debt for
long.

> ❝As a well-spent day brings
> happy sleep, so life well used
> brings happy death.❞
>
> *Leonardo da Vinci*

Busy mind

One of the main obstacles to getting off to sleep is having a busy mind. If you are constantly going over problems in your mind, your thinking and judgement become clouded, but when you mentally relax and switch off your conscious thoughts, you take back control.

As well as the techniques in Chapter 9: Overcoming the Worries that Keep Us Awake, try the hypnosis below.

Calming your mind technique

This technique is fantastic in helping you to wind down before sleep. Use it 30 minutes before you go to bed and you will sleep like a baby! If you have a lot going on and feel mentally stressed, it will help to calm your mind and alleviate tension. It could be categorised as more of a meditation than self-hypnosis, as it has a kind of higher consciousness flavour to it. However, the label is unimportant; what does matter is that you embrace it and put your feelings into it so that you heighten your sensitivity and become centred and deeply relaxed.

You can use this technique for 20 or 30 minutes at a time. You will be amazed at how relaxed you are afterwards. You may even find it helps you to feel more creative or gives you greater clarity. Remember that you have so many resources in your unconscious mind. This is where your real talents and creativity lie, and to get to them, you have to suspend all intellectual thought and bypass your analytical, conscious mind. This is why switching off your conscious mind is so important.

Read through the instructions below a few times until you know what to do and then practise this whenever you need to quieten your mind before you go to sleep.

When you get into a deeply relaxed mental state during this meditation, you will also be experiencing the state of waking hypnosis, in which you are in a deep trance but have your eyes open.

Go to a quiet room where there are no distractions. Light a candle and place it in front of you. Turn off all lights so the only light is from the candle's flame.

Sit comfortably in front of the candle and focus on the flickering flame. Watch the movement of the flame and begin to breathe very slowly and deeply in through your nose and out through your mouth.

Make each circular breath long and deep, and clear away any thoughts so your mind becomes still and centred. Don't worry if you get the odd unwanted thought. Just centre your mind again and allow the thought to drift away. Focus on your breathing and the stillness of the moment, and continue your slow, deep circular breathing.

Keep your eyes on the flame and remain centred and focused. Be in the here and now and accept everything as it is. With every slow, deep breath allow yourself to relax even more and focus your mind only on the flame. Watch the unique movements of the flame and notice its colour changing.

You can stay in this pleasant state for as long as you like. There is no ideal time limit, so do whatever feels right for you at the time. When you practise this mental workout, focus on nothing but clearing your mind and staying centred. Don't underestimate the power of this simple technique, as it is a great way of completely calming your mind.

When you have finished, blow out the candle and close your eyes. Remain in a centred state and avoid intellectual thought or analysis. After a minute or so, you can go to bed and sleep easily.

Chapter 7

THE SLEEP WELL PROGRAMME – STEPS 2, 3 AND 4

Step 2: The ultimate hydration remedy to cure sleep problems

Far too many people are dehydrated, which can lead to a multitude of problems, including sleep deprivation. Some studies show that dehydration can even lead to various degrees of anxiety and depression, and that drinking more water can alleviate these symptoms. Drinking lots of water should be something that you make a permanent habit even after you establish a good sleep pattern.

We need to drink around six pints of water a day to avoid our cells becoming dehydrated. It is also important to drink good-quality fresh mineral water, so avoid tap water as most tap water is full of impurities and chemicals. The best water filter you can buy to purify your tap water is a five-stage reverse-osmosis filter. These can be costly and bulky, but investing in your health is always a wise move. If your budget doesn't stretch to an all-singing-all-dancing water filter, buy one that suits your budget.

From now on, get into the habit of drinking a pint of fresh water when you wake and then five more throughout the day. Water with a slice of lemon is a good cleanser and refresher first thing in the morning. Avoid drinking your last pint of water too late so that you don't wake up to go to the loo in the night.

When you can get into the habit of drinking six pints a day, you will notice many benefits. Drinking fresh water helps to flush away toxins, improves your skin complexion, helps with digestion and can replace the need for snacking in between meals. The following visualisation technique will help you create a new habit of drinking lots of water each day.

☽ Loving the Taste of Pure ☽ Fresh Water technique

This technique will help you to programme your mind to really enjoy drinking lots of fresh water. Visualising drinking water and affirming that you love pure fresh water will help you create a new healthy habit that will benefit you in so many ways.

Close your eyes and take a few slow, deep breaths. Centre your mind and repeat the following affirmation to yourself over and over in a slow, rhythmical chant:

I love the taste of pure fresh water.

As you affirm this, imagine the crystal-clear water pouring into your mouth, bringing you a strong feeling of refreshment. Taste the water in your mouth and really enjoy the feeling of drinking it.

After the first time you use this technique, drink a fresh glass of bottled or filtered water and you will notice how good it tastes.

From now on, whenever you drink water, affirm to yourself silently 'I love the taste of pure fresh water.' Say it over and over, and feel good as you say it. Each time you drink water, imagine the water trickling down your throat and into your system, revitalising and refreshing you.

Use this water visualisation often and you will be well on the way to creating a very healthy habit that will last you a lifetime.

Step 3: The ultimate healthy-eating remedy to cure sleep problems

A healthy diet is important for many things, including sleep. If your diet is good and you avoid eating late, you will be taking another big step towards your goal of regular healthy sleep at night.

Anything that your body can digest easily, like fruit, will not cause you too much restlessness at night, but certain foods and drinks are not conducive to good sleep. Most of this is fairly obvious – any food or drink that stimulates the body should be avoided well before bedtime. Processed foods that are hard for the body to digest should not be eaten late in the day, or ideally at any time.

Too much salt is said to interfere with a restful sleep and so your salt intake should be minimised. Sugar is much the same; in fact, there is not a single nutritional benefit from eating processed sugar, which is added to so many food products nowadays. Why not eliminate it from your diet completely? I did years ago and don't miss it at all.

It is also wise to avoid replacing sugar with artificial sweeteners as they can be even worse for your health than processed sugar. So cross off your shopping lists any products that are labelled 'sugar-free', 'low sugar' or 'diet', as the manufacturers will have added artificial sweeteners that often include the highly unpleasant aspartame and saccharine, which also have stimulating properties. If ever you want to sweeten something, add a little organic honey instead.

You should also cut down or avoid completely white flour products, tea, coffee, chocolate, cola and fizzy sugar drinks in general, alcohol, fatty foods, fried foods and foods containing additives. A balanced healthy diet will go a long way in helping you to sleep well at night.

☽ Sleep tip – eat slowly

Make a habit of eating slowly and be conscious of your food as you eat. By eating slowly and chewing your food well, you will satisfy your taste buds more completely, enabling you to feel full quickly. This will assist you with any weight issues, and importantly, it also helps your body to digest the food more easily, which will help you to sleep better.

Eat consciously and healthily, and from now on make your meals last longer.

'But I couldn't give up coffee and chocolate!' I hear you say. Well, actually, you could, if you chose to. It is simply a matter of programming your mind. With most young people, their first experience of alcohol or smoking is usually unpleasant, but often peer pressure and the desire to be grown-up drive them to overcome any initial dislike. They literally train their minds to enjoy the stuff and in no time they are hooked and alcohol and/or smoking becomes part of their lives.

Breaking free of unwanted habits is easy with hypnosis, as it is an instant way of reprogramming your mind. Coffee and chocolate do very little for you other than slow your metabolism, make you put on weight and add to sleep problems, as they have a stimulating effect. So if you could get rid of them from your diet for ever and genuinely not miss them, would you go for that? It's a no-brainer, as you have nothing to lose and everything to gain. Think of the fact that your sleep patterns are far more important than eating chocolate or drinking coffee.

〉 Eradicating Unhealthy 〉 Food or Drinks technique

This technique is excellent for helping you to banish coffee or chocolate, which I am using as examples of food and drink that play a part in sleep problems, but you can use the technique to get rid of any food or drink from your diet. Your sleep is of paramount importance and you must avoid food and drinks that hinder it.

Think of a **single** unhealthy or fattening food or drink that you would like to eradicate from your diet now.

Close your eyes and take a few slow, deep breaths and allow your mind to clear. Take a moment to go inside yourself and totally relax. When you are ready, imagine a plate full of the most putrid, rotting fish or maggots or something similar that is repulsive to you. It has to be something you intensely dislike.

See this picture in your mind's eye and connect with the revolting smell of the fish. Hold back from gagging, but make this image smell very real. Take a moment to do this.

When you have a clear picture and have imagined

the foul smell, bring in the food or drink you want to erase from your diet and mix it up with the rotting fish. If it is chocolate, imagine the chocolate all over the fish, making an even more disgusting smell. If it is coffee or a fizzy drink, imagine one of the fish inside a cup of coffee or a glass of pop.

Be creative with this part of the technique; the more vivid you can make this image, the more powerful it will be. Allow a few minutes to digest this disgusting image and odour, and then allow your mind to become blank. Take a few slow breaths, before slowly counting to three and opening your eyes.

Do this a number of times over the next few days. After this time, you will feel completely different about the food or drink that you mixed up with the rotting fish. You will lose any desire for that food or drink, or you may even find it repulsive.

You can use this technique to systematically eradicate any other junk foods and drinks from your diet. Focus on eliminating **one thing at a time** and make sure you have lost all desire for it before moving on to the next item you want to eradicate.

Step 4: The ultimate exercise remedy to cure sleep problems

While exercise alone will not solve all sleep problems, it is another factor that will help you improve your quality of sleep. Studies show that people who exercise at least a couple of times a week are less likely to suffer from sleep disorders. Studies at the Netherlands Institute for Brain Research found that exercise helped elderly people to improve their quality of sleep by reducing the disturbances in their circadian rhythms. They also found that men in their seventies who exercised in the day slept better than those who didn't exercise frequently. So it is a good idea to make a habit of exercising more each day so that you find it easier to sleep at night.

One note of caution, though: avoid vigorous exercise too near to bedtime, as this will have a stimulating effect that is obviously detrimental to getting to sleep. If you do participate in strenuous exercise, make sure it is at least three hours before your bedtime. You should ideally practise more strenuous exercise earlier in the day, and later on in the day do a more gentle form of exercise, like yoga, which helps you to wind down. In fact, yoga is an ideal de-stress workout, and even if you are unable to join a class, it is well worth learning a few basic poses from the many DVDs on the market or videos available online. Yoga an hour before bedtime will help you release tension and physically prepare for sleep.

For those of you who want to delve into yoga more deeply, the specific yoga poses that can help with insomnia are shirshasana, sarvangasana, paschimottanasana, uttanasana, viparit karni and shavasana.

To improve your fitness levels in the long term, you must come from a mindset that tells you you are creating a new holistic, healthy lifestyle. So many people initially build a strong resolve to get fit only to give up after three months and drift back to their old unhealthy ways. Fitness clubs can happily oversell memberships because they know that 80 per cent of people who join stop going after three months. If all members of any given gym turned up at once, they would not be able to cope.

If you need additional help in the area of exercise motivation and healthy eating, I have produced dedicated hypnosis audio recordings that cover these topics. You will find information in the Further Resources section on page 175. I have created a hypnosis audio from the following technique, which also works well as a self-hypnosis technique.

⟋ℰ⟍ **Exercise tip**

To improve your level of physical fitness, you must become more active. You can start by simply walking more. It is so easy to drive everywhere these days, but if you get the opportunity, walk instead. For example, don't get frustrated if you can't park right outside the restaur-ant or shop you visit; park a few hundred metres away and walk. Look at the lack of parking spaces as an opportunity to get a little exercise. It is nice to have a short walk after leaving a restaurant, as it will help you to digest your meal and burn a few calories. Another tip is to avoid escalators and elevators, and always use the stairs if you can.

When you incorporate these ideas into your daily life, they become habits that you get into and enjoy. They also cost you very little time and become part of your everyday approach to fitness. There is always another way of viewing things, and if you reframe your attitude towards exercise, you will never again be disappointed because an elevator is not working or you can't find a parking space.

Work on your fitness slowly by doing a little each day and building up to a level that feels good for you.

) Learning to Love Exercise) technique

If you want to become more active but have lacked motivation in the past, the following technique will help you to build a strong inner desire to exercise regularly.

Stop at this point and read through the text below a few times until you are familiar with the technique. The key to getting the best out of this technique is to **connect a strong feeling of pleasure and enjoyment to exercise.** Once you have a grasp of the technique, practise it often so that your desire to exercise and become more active on a daily basis is second nature.

Don't worry if you feel you're not going very deep into a trance in this exercise, or any other. Even if you close your eyes and simply visualise and affirm, you will still make a big difference. The important thing is to do this regularly so that you compound the new images and affirmations. Always remember this: affirmations and visualisations are a remark-ably effective re-programming method even in the lightest trance states.

Go to a quiet, darkened room where there are no distractions. Take a moment to get in a comfortable position, close your eyes and focus your attention on your breathing. Begin to breathe very slowly and deeply in through your nose and out through your mouth. Make each breath long and deep. Feel your ribcage expand as you breathe in. Continue this for a short while until all the tension disappears from your body and you feel relaxed.

Continue to breathe slowly and deeply in a steady, rhythmical breathing pattern, and when you reach the top of your breath, hold it for three seconds: one…two…three. Then silently and mentally count to five on every out-breath: one…two…three…four…five. Relax more and more with every slow out-breath.

Now I want you to practise a more instant way of going into a trance. Slowly and steadily count from one to three either silently or out loud: one…two…three. When you reach the number three, say to yourself, 'I will become ten times more deeply relaxed.' You will go ten times deeper inside that powerful part of yourself where your true potential lies: your creativity, your courage, and your self-belief. At the very point you reach the number three, go deep down into a very relaxed state. So ready? One…two…three. Go there now. More deeply relaxed than you've been in a long time. Every cell in your mind, body and spirit now resonates with positive energy. Take a short while to connect with this still, centred feeling.

If you don't master this the first time, don't worry as it may take practice before you can go into a deep trance very quickly. If you prefer, you can use one of the other methods described in this book.

Now to the visualisation part. Imagine yourself participating in exercise and feel yourself really enjoying it. It is important to use your feelings here so that you anchor a strong sense of enjoyment into your unconscious mind. Maybe visualise yourself working out at the gym, practising yoga, playing tennis, cycling, jogging or whatever works for you. As you see yourself doing one or more activity, connect with a feeling of great pleasure and enjoyment. Make the visualisation clear and use all of your five senses to create a realistic mental image. Take a little time to do this and let your imagination go.

After you have visualised, I want you to repeat the following affirmations to yourself in the present tense. Say each affirmation ten times or more in a rhythmical way, almost like a slow, steady chant. Say your affirmations with real feeling and emotion. Imagine every part of you repeating the affirmations with complete conviction and self-belief. Draw the phrases deep inside you as you say them.

I love to exercise and keep fit.

I go beyond old limitations and draw out my true potential.

I deserve to be fit and healthy.

I always sleep well after exercising.

You can even state the affirmations as a soundtrack to your visualisation when you get the hang of it. Once you have stated and focused on your affirmations, you can compound these new beliefs by the counting method. Once again, count from one to three. This time, when you reach the number three, affirm that these positive new beliefs will root ten times more deeply into your unconscious mind and that the positive feelings will grow ten times stronger. Feel yourself drawing all your new beliefs deeply into your inner consciousness. Every cell in your mind, body and spirit is resonating with positive energy now. Take a moment to enjoy this feeling and to accept every new belief as a reality.

When you are ready, slowly count from one to ten, open your eyes and come back to full waking consciousness.

☯ Sleep Well Programme case study

A client once came to me to help cure his chronic insomnia. He had tried many solutions in the past, but none had been completely effective. He had even tried self-hypnosis, and although it had improved his sleep, it was still not perfect. It transpired that his bedroom resembled an entertainment centre, and after a little persuasion he cleared out the TV, stereo and PC equipment. We also worked on improving his diet and avoiding stimulating food and drinks at night. The combination of these changes and the personalised hypnotherapy sessions improved his sleep to the point where he could sleep for most of the night most of the time. Before, his sleep had been so bad that if he slept for two hours, he considered this to be a good night.

This case study highlights the need for a holistic approach. The combination of lifestyle changes, one-to-one sessions and the continued use of self-hypnosis helped to cure this gent of his chronic insomnia...naturally!

Chapter 8

THE SLEEP WELL PROGRAMME – STEPS 5 AND 6

Step 5: The ultimate natural remedies to cure sleep problems

Natural solutions free of side-effects and dependency have to be the best option for overcoming insomnia. Recent research has shown that cognitive behaviour therapy can be more effective than medication in controlling insomnia. In this therapy, patients are taught improved sleep habits and relieved of counter-productive assumptions about sleep. This, combined with the mental and physical relaxation elements of hypnotherapy, would provide most people with the ideal solution for sleep disorders.

Relaxation techniques used in **self-hypnosis** and **meditation** are a great aid to restful, deep sleep. The more a person is both mentally and physically relaxed, the greater their chances will be of getting a good night's sleep. This is because both techniques slow brainwaves and relax the mind and body. When you are in a state of deep self-hypnosis or meditation, it is an easy transition to then fall asleep, which leads to a deeper, more restful sleep.

Slow-paced relaxation music and **sound effects** created in certain keys can also help to create a state of relaxation ideal for restful sleep. This is something I use on my hypnosis audio with this book – the background sound effects have been created in certain keys and frequencies that aid deep relaxation.

Thiamine, also known as **vitamin B**, can be helpful in the treatment of insomnia as it is vital for strong, healthy nerves. A body lacking in thiamine will find it difficult to relax and sleep easily. Natural sources of this vitamin are found in wholegrain cereals, pulses and nuts. A good-quality vitamin-B supplement would also suffice; not all vitamins are of the same standard, so seek out a manufacturer of the highest quality. It is also important to note that if you do take vitamins on a daily basis, you must avoid taking any before bedtime, as vitamins take time to digest and can stimulate your body.

Pomegranates are believed to contain natural properties that help insomniacs sleep, and **lettuce** can also be included in the treatment of insomnia as it contains a sleep-inducing substance called lactucarium. **Milk sweetened with honey** is also said to act as a relaxant, although I'm not a fan of milk as it is often loaded with additives and growth hormones. Instead, I would recommend two teaspoons of **organic honey** in a large cup of water four hours before going to bed. Honey is said to have a hypnotic action and induces a sound sleep.

Chamomile tea and **aniseed tea** are other possibilities you may want to look at in your quest for good sleep. Chamomile tea can be bought in most health stores and supermarkets, and aniseed tea can be made by adding a teaspoon of aniseed to boiling water. The water should be covered with a lid and allowed to simmer for 15 minutes. It should then be strained into a cup. The tea may be sweetened with honey and taken after your last meal.

☽ Sleep tip – eliminate caffeine

Did you know that the caffeine from coffee and tea consumption stays in your system for many hours? So avoid tea or coffee in the evening. Better still, switch to drinking decaffeinated tea or coffee or the herbal teas.

Herbs such as chamomile, lavender, hops, valerian, rauwolfia and passion flower have natural sedative effects. For insomnia, try taking a warm bath in the evening with any of the natural oil-based herbs mentioned above.

Aromatherapy is a wonderful way of relaxing the mind and body, and relieving stress. Aromatherapy oils including jasmine and lavender may contain natural properties that lead to a state of restfulness. Reflexology can also help relieve stress and so help with sleep problems.

Traditional Chinese medicine that can help with sleep problems includes acupuncture, dietary and lifestyle analysis and herbology. The goal is to resolve the root cause of the sleep problem.

Specific forms of **Buddhist meditation** can also help. In the Buddhist tradition, people suffering from insomnia or nightmares may be advised to meditate on 'loving kindness'. This practice of generating a feeling of love and goodwill is claimed to have a soothing, calming effect on the mind and body. This is claimed to stem partly from the creation of relaxing, positive thoughts and feelings, and partly from the pacification of negative ones.

Homeopathy is another alternative treatment that may offer solutions for some sleep problems. Homeopathic remedies treat like with like and contain very small amounts of the active ingredient. The nature and root causes of a patient's sleeplessness are an integral part of homeopathic treatment, so it is wise to seek out a qualified homeopath for diagnosis. Here are some of the homeopathic remedies used to treat insomnia:

- **Pulsatilla** can help calm the mind from repetitive thoughts. It is also used to treat excesses of emotion, mood swings and temper tantrums.

- **Coffea**, from the coffee bush, is generally thought of as a stimulant; in homeopathy, however, its properties are used in minute amounts to ease the way to sleep when excitement arises after hearing good or bad news.

- **Nux vomica** can help with indigestion-related sleeplessness. It is also a popular hangover remedy and is often used to counteract the effects of sleeplessness caused by caffeine, alcohol or drugs.

Natural remedy checklist

1 Try meditation, Buddhist meditation and relaxation techniques.

2 Take a daily vitamin B supplement.

3 Increase your intake of pomegranates, lettuce, honey in warm water, chamomile tea and aniseed tea.

4 Try regular herbal treatments such as chamomile, lavender, hops, valerian, rauwolfia and passion flower.

5 Consider using alternative treatments such as aromatherapy, reflexology, herbology, acupuncture and homeopathy.

Step 6: The ultimate self-hypnosis remedy to cure sleep problems

The following self-hypnosis technique is an in-depth guide to self-hypnosis for alleviating sleep problems. It will help you to relax your mind and body in preparation for a good night's sleep. When you use self-hypnosis or you meditate, you allow your mind to rest and recuperate. This technique is slightly longer than the others in this book and will help you reach even deeper levels of mental and physical relaxation.

It will also work wonders in calming your mind and alleviating stress. If you are constantly going over problems in your mind, your thinking and judgement become clouded. This technique helps free you from these problems. Once you get the hang of it, you will be amazed at how good you feel in the morning.

Stop at this point and read the script through a few times until you know what to do and then practise this technique every night before you go to sleep – unless you prefer to use the recording, that is. You can use the audio most nights, then use this self-hypnosis technique as and when the mood takes you. Use whatever combination works best for you.

You will find that the more you practise self-hypnosis, the deeper into a trance you will go each time, and the better you will get at de-stressing your mind.

〉 Basic Breathing technique 〉

When you are lying down in bed and ready for sleep, begin by telling yourself silently that you are going to use self-hypnosis to go to sleep.

Close your eyes and begin to breathe very slowly and deeply in through your nose and out through your mouth. Make each circular breath long and deep, and at the top of your breath, hold it for three seconds, then count to five on every out-breath. As you breathe out, imagine you are breathing away any nervous tension left in your body.

If you wish, you can also say the word 'relax' on every out-breath. Continue this breathing pattern ten or more times, or as long as it takes for you to feel completely relaxed.

☽ Diaphragmatic Breathing ☽ technique

Once you get the hang of the Basic Breathing technique, you can add the Diaphragmatic Breathing technique. Make sure that you breathe from your diaphragm (lower chest and stomach area) and not from the upper chest. Watch what happens to your body as you breathe. If you are breathing properly, your stomach will go out as you breathe in and will go in as you breathe out. This can take a little practice if you are unused to diaphragmatic breathing.

》 Mind-emptying 》 technique

Allow your mind to go completely blank. Don't worry if you still get unwanted thoughts drifting into your mind; tell yourself not to fight them, as they will soon drift away again. Every time you get an unwanted thought, imagine a large red stop sign. As soon as you see the stop sign, imagine the thought disappearing and your mind becoming clear.

Another thought-clearing technique is to imagine a large computer screen full of data that becomes blank by hitting a keypad. Imagine that by pressing a keypad, you can clear your mind. Another method is to imagine you are looking up at the sky on a pleasant summer's day. You notice a few small clouds that drift across the sky and then fade away. Eventually all of the clouds have drifted away and the sky is clear. Imagine your conscious thoughts are like clouds that fade away. Use whatever method works for you.

☽ Relaxing Your Body ☽ technique

Now you can relax your body. Imagine every muscle from the top of your head to the tips of your toes completely relaxing. You can start at the top and systematically work your way down to your toes. Imagine your eyelids have become heavy and tired, and any tension in your forehead is disappearing. All the muscles there are becoming loose and relaxed.

Continue this pattern and imagine all the muscles relaxing in your jaw, neck, shoulders, back, arms and legs. Imagine the relaxation spreading down through your body, letting go of any tightness or tension in the muscles. You can visualise the muscles relaxing, and spend extra time relaxing any part of your body that holds most tension. Allow the outside world to fade into the background and continue your journey into your inner world.

❱❱ Utilising the trance state ❱❱ with affirmations

When you have finished your body relaxation and you are completely relaxed from head to toe, you can repeat the following affirmations. It is important you only say them word for word as they are below.

When you repeat these affirmations, imagine every part of you absorbing the phrases with real belief, and use your feelings and emotions to supercharge them so that every cell in your mind and body resonates with each positive affirmation.

I sleep easily at night.

I feel deeply relaxed.

I feel calm and centred.

I love to sleep at night.

At this point, you can allow yourself to drift off into a deep, natural sleep from which you will wake feeling refreshed.

Congratulations! You have now reached the end of the Sleep Well Programme, which forms the foundation for tackling most sleep problems. In Section 3: More Sleep Solutions, we will look in more detail at overcoming stress and anxiety, which are the source of many people's sleep problems, and will also offer solutions for some of the more unusual causes of sleepless nights.

☯ Golden Sleep Rule

5. Cut out stimulants and reduce salt intake.

Avoid stimulating food and drinks such as white flour products, sugar, tea, coffee, chocolate, cola and fizzy drinks in general, alcohol, fatty foods, fried foods and foods containing additives. Also minimise your salt intake.

SECTION 3

MORE SLEEP SOLUTIONS

Chapter 9

OVERCOMING THE WORRIES THAT KEEP US AWAKE

No more tossing and turning at night

Anxiety and worry cause many people sleepless nights, but it really doesn't have to be this way. Worrying in bed is a complete waste of time. All it will do is stimulate your intellect and keep you awake. If you use the hypnosis techniques in this chapter, you need never again lie in bed at night and allow your conscious mind to churn over problems.

☽ Clearing Your Mind ☽ technique

This self-hypnosis technique is ideal if you have lots of worries that have been playing on your mind. It will allow your creative mind to find solutions to problems, while at the same time stilling your conscious mind and preparing for sleep.

Close your eyes and begin to breathe very slowly and deeply in through your nose and out through your mouth. Make each circular breath long and deep, and breathe away any tension with every slow out-breath. Allow the chatter of your mind to quieten and aim to let your mind go blank. An empty mind is key in this technique, so spend time getting your mind to be still. Don't worry if you still get unwanted thoughts; just allow them to drift away again.

After 15 minutes or so, when you feel pleasantly relaxed and your mind is very still, begin to accept that your unconscious mind will find a solution to this problem. Avoid thinking about the actual problem itself or even thinking of a solution, as that will only stimulate your intellect. If at any time you feel yourself intellectualising, then allow your mind to go blank and take a few slow, deep breaths to return to that centred space.

Your aim is simply to focus on your creative mind's ability to find solutions and affirm that it will – as though you are programming your mind to deliver a solution to you without thinking about the problem itself.

When you are in that deeply relaxed, still space, you can also repeat one or more of the affirmations below:

A solution will soon come to me at exactly the right time.

My creative mind will give me the answer.

I trust in my own judgement.

When using affirmations, remember to put your feelings into them, as this makes them stronger and anchors them more deeply in your unconscious mind. So really feel each statement is a reality as you affirm it. You can also add your own affirmations, but make sure they are along the same lines as these and that they are not mentioning the problem itself.

After affirming to yourself, you can let go and go to sleep with the knowledge that your unconscious mind will find a solution to your problem. This may materialise in the form of a new line of thought the next day, or you may suddenly experience some clarity out of the blue.

〉 Relaxing Your Mind With 〉 Colour technique

This is another great technique to help you when your body is exhausted but your mind is racing and you are finding it difficult to wind down.

Allow 20 minutes before you go to sleep. You can use this technique in bed or before you actually get into bed. Just make sure you begin 20 minutes or so before you actually want to go to sleep.

Get into a comfortable position, then close your eyes and begin to breathe very slowly and deeply in through your nose and out through your mouth. Make each circular breath a little longer and deeper than the last, and breathe away any tension with every slow out-breath. Continue to centre yourself for about five or ten minutes, until your mind is still and quiet, and you feel nicely relaxed.

Then imagine a blue light coming up through the soles of your feet, slowly filling your body in the same way a tall glass would fill with water. Feel the blue light relaxing you and calming your mind further. Once the blue light reaches the top of your

head and you are immersed in this light, just allow
yourself to bathe in the healing colour for a while.
Allow yourself to become more and more relaxed at
this point, and when you are ready, you can go into a
deep, peaceful sleep.

Blue is a very calming colour, and this simple visualisation is a great way to prepare yourself for sleep.

Worrying about the future

If you worry about something in the future when you
lie in bed at night, this will not help you sleep. It could
be that you have an upcoming job interview, a speech to
make, a public performance or an important meeting.
Any future event that is giving you sleepless nights
can be remedied by flipping your mind out of constant
worry and stress, and into a far more productive state
that will help you on the big day.

When all you do is worry about a future event, you
are programming your mind with fear, which it will
respond to at the time of the future event. I have seen
highly capable, intelligent people blow big opportunities because of the anxiety that they created around an

event. You see it all the time on TV talent shows, when skilled would-be singers crumble when they are asked to perform under pressure. When I see this, I always wish I could help them, as it is really so easy to overcome stage fright.

The very best way to conquer the worry of dealing with pressured situations is to visualise the future event and create an entirely positive scenario using all of your senses and as much creativity as possible. This way, you will set yourself up to succeed by creating a peak-performance state at the time when you need it most. Positive programming is something that most top sportspeople use, as do many people who are successful in their careers.

The technique below is invaluable in helping you to be at your best. It works so effectively because of a key ingredient in mind programming – the human mind doesn't distinguish between what is real and what is imagined. So when you create a visualisation, your mind will accept it as a reality. Needless to say, avoiding negative scenarios and regularly creating positive visualisations can help you in a multitude of ways. We are all blessed with an ability to imagine, and when we learn how to harness the power of our imagination, we can achieve practically anything.

☽ Future Event Visualisation ☽ technique

This is the perfect technique to get you into a peak-performance state. It will also help you to overcome anxiety in the kind of pressured situations we all face at different times. If the event that is causing you sleepless nights is something like a flight and you are anxious about flying or you have a big exam, driving test, interview, public performance, speech or whatever, it is good to use this technique every night for two weeks before the big day. Think of it as though you are programming yourself to succeed and every time you do this you strengthen the new pattern. Even if you are out on a date the next day or you have an important meeting in the morning, you can use this the night before to prepare yourself in the best possible way.

Go to bed 30 minutes earlier than usual. Get yourself comfortable, close your eyes and focus your attention on your breathing technique. Allow your mind and body to relax.

Once you are deeply relaxed and your mind is still, begin to imagine the future situation that is keeping you awake at night and visualise it in a positive light. See it exactly how you want it to be. Imagine you are performing to the best of your ability and are at your absolute best. You are strong, confident, in control, calm and secure. Remember you are programming your mind, which will believe and accept what you are visualising without question. The more positive you make the visualisation, the better you will be on the big day.

Now make the pictures bigger and brighter, and supercharge the pictures by putting your feelings into them. Feel a surge of confidence and self-belief as you run the images in your mind. Believe on every level you are succeeding. Accept this belief unconditionally. Take a moment to enjoy the successful scenario. As you do so, the feelings and images will sink deeply into your unconscious mind and become part of your inner reality. Your unconscious mind will then accept this positive future event as real.

Now you can go to sleep knowing that there is nothing to worry about, as you have just programmed your mind in a very positive way.

Focus on a **single goal** each night, and if this was something that had been causing you a lot of sleeplessness, use the technique repeatedly night after night with this single goal in mind. Always work on one thing at a time. The key is to use your feelings and make the events as real as you can. Really *feeling* it is crucial!

This Future Event Visualisation technique will help you work towards any goal successfully. You can even use it for your future more generally, so that you see yourself in several years' time looking happy, healthy and abundant, with everything as you want it to be. Work on that visualisation for a while and just see how things begin to change for you!

Creating profoundly positive beliefs about your future on a deep, unconscious level can help you in many subtle ways. It can help you to become more intuitive, so you automatically make many more good decisions than bad ones.

Practise this technique often. It is so much more productive than lying awake at night and worrying.

Worrying about money

One of the biggest causes of worry and sleepless nights in this day and age is financial stress. However, worrying about money is not the exclusive pastime of people who are broke; it is also something that wealthy people often indulge in. Those without money tend to worry about not having enough, and those with it tend to worry

☽ Sleep tip – programming your computer

Think of your mind as being like a computer: what you put in will come back out. The human mind is exactly like that, so from now on you must *never* vocally or internally say or even think negative things about yourself. I know this is not always easy if you have had a lifetime of negative conditioning and your self-esteem is low, but you need to start afresh from this moment on.

By programming your computer with positive beliefs about yourself and avoiding negative self-talk, over time you will build confidence and self-esteem. It is a case of fake it until you make it.

about maintaining the standard of living they've become used to.

I would imagine even the super-rich have sleepless nights worrying about controlling their empires. Apparently, when Roman Abramovich got divorced, he had to pay his ex-wife £2.5 billion, which no doubt gave him a few sleepless nights.

I'm being a little tongue in cheek here, but it does show how we are all capable of losing sleep over money worries, regardless of our financial position. The reason we worry so much about money is because it is linked to security, which is a fundamental human need.

Worrying about money is probably one of the worst things you can do, as by creating fear, you will be blocking any natural abundance. Instead of tossing and turning at night and worrying about paying bills or how to keep up the mortgage payments, simply reframe your thinking so that you focus your mind on abundance. When you give your attention to creating abundance, you will worry less and build up a new stream of creative thinking.

By focusing on abundance, you naturally become more receptive to it. I speak as a person who was terminally skint for an insufferably long time and who then became reasonably abundant in a short space of time. This dramatic change happened when I woke up to the realisation that creating abundance starts with a mindset that is open and prepared to accept success and abundance. Too many people believe only others get rich or that there is a spiritual virtue in struggle and hardship. Not true. I've done the old struggle and hardship bit and it didn't elevate my spiritual self in the slightest. I moaned a lot instead!

It is a positive thing to aim to be abundant because when you are, you can experience life more fully through travel and other opportunities afforded by an increase in income. The following technique should be used any time that financial concerns are affecting your sleep.

☽ Creating More ☽ Abundance technique

You can use this technique before bedtime or at any time of the day or night. If you use this technique when you are in bed at night, you can drift off to sleep after repeating the affirmations. If you are using it during the day and you need to wake up feeling refreshed and alert, simply count slowly from one to ten, becoming more awake with each number. At eight, open your eyes, and at ten, come back to full waking consciousness.

You will spend much less time worrying about money when you get into a habit of using this technique and repeating the affirmations regularly. Instead, your energy will be focused on creating abundance by seeing more opportunities around you.

Get in a comfortable position, close your eyes and focus your attention on your breathing. Then begin breathing slowly and deeply in through your nose and out through your mouth. Breathe away any tension left in your body with every slow out-breath and allow yourself to relax more and more. Continue this breathing pattern a dozen or more times and clear away any unwanted thoughts so that your mind becomes still and quiet. Don't worry if you get the odd unwanted thought. Just focus on the stillness of the moment.

Now, as you lie there in this stillness, imagine yourself in a very abundant position. Imagine that you are surrounded by opportunities and that you find it easy to create success in your life. See yourself with boundless enthusiasm and full of new ideas.

You can take things a step further and imagine your dream lifestyle with you living in your dream home and ideal car, and doing work that you love and enjoy that generates so much abundance. Make the visualisation whatever you want it to be.

When you create these pictures, it is crucially important to make the visualisation in the present tense and not to put a limit on your success. The more you feel it and believe it, the more effective it will be. Make your visualisation bright, colourful and vivid.

When you are ready, repeat the following magical affirmations to yourself over and over again. Say them to yourself slowly and deliberately, as though you are drawing them deeply inside you.

I am always in the right place at the right time.

Abundance flows freely and naturally to me.

All of my needs are constantly met.

I have found these affirmations to be particularly effective. As always, when you state these phrases, really believe they are a reality. Put your feelings into each phrase and repeat the affirmations like a steady mantra. Once you get used to the sequence, you can even repeat them in your daily life.

Chapter 10

ELIMINATING THE HIDDEN CAUSES OF POOR SLEEP

What effect do electromagnetic fields have on sleep?

As we saw in Step 1 of the Sleep Well Programme, electromagnetic fields are frequencies given off by all electrical devices from electric alarm clocks to plasma TVs. Some electrical devices, such as wireless technology and mobile phones, will put out a stronger EMF than others. Bedside lamps and electric alarm clocks will emit low levels of EMFs, but if you want to banish all EMFs from your bedroom, use a non-electric, old-fashioned, wind-up alarm clock.

Even being subjected to EMFs *before* you go to bed can affect your sleep. At the Brain Sciences Institute at Swinburne University of Technology in Australia, 50 participants were exposed to EMFs from mobile phones for 30 minutes prior to sleep. Results showed a decrease in rapid eye movement during the initial part of sleep following EMF exposure. These results are evidence that EMF exposure even before going to sleep is likely to disrupt sleep patterns.

Another study, at the Institute of Pharmacology and Toxicology at the University of Zurich, showed that the use of mobile phones 30 minutes before sleep altered brainwaves, affecting sleep patterns adversely.

There are many other studies showing that EMFs can disrupt sleep patterns, and the bottom line is that if you want to improve your sleep patterns, removing all EMFs from your bedroom is a must. So even if you have a groovy plasma on your bedroom wall, it has to go – as do *any* hi-fis, computer equipment or telephones. Your sleep is too important. You must also avoid using computers, mobile phones or any device with a strong EMF close to bedtime.

☽ Sleep tip – the best alarm clock

As most of us are governed by time, an alarm clock is essential. However, traditional alarm clocks are designed to wake us instantly with a load of noise. From the beginning of time, humans have learned to respond to the rising dawn by waking up gradually. A sudden noise is the worst possible way to wake, even if you have become conditioned to it. This way of waking can leave you feeling weary and irritable all day.

The solution is to buy a natural daylight alarm clock, which gives the effect of sunset and sunrise by slowly turning off at night and slowly coming on in the morning. These ingenious alarm clocks help us to wake in a much more natural way. Gradually waking at the onset of daylight also helps our internal body clock to synchronise. They are particularly effective during the winter months, when the days are shortest and the body is exposed to the least amount of natural light.

Clinical studies at the National Institute of Health in the US indicate that waking to light has been known to help people with seasonal affective disorder (SAD), various forms of depression and sleep disorders. It increased their daytime energy, limited winter weight gain and allowed them to wake up more easily.

These clocks also simulate sunset, which gives your body the signal to wind down and go to sleep. Some manufacturers even produce a version of these clocks for toddlers and babies.

A Google search under 'natural daylight alarm clocks' will help you to locate suppliers.

⟩ Degaussing technique ⟩

Every living organism has an electromagnetic field, including human beings. Many believe that overexposure to EMFs from technological devices can create a kind of electrical smog and clog our own electromagnetic fields. This can manifest in feelings of restlessness, listlessness, not being able to unwind, restless leg syndrome, feeling mentally scattered and being unable to sleep. It can also have the effect of leaving you feeling addicted to a computer or games device even when you don't really want to use them any more.

Practitioners of the alternative therapy of health kinesiology use a technique called degaussing to clear the electrical smog that accumulates in our EMF. Health kinesiologists say that in the same way that your skin gets dirty and needs cleaning so does your EMF or aura. The technique seems a little unusual, but if you use the computer a lot and you have any of the feelings described above, then give it a try. Use it after excessive exposure to technology devices. You will soon know if it helps you to wind down more easily and be better prepared for sleep.

For this technique, you need something with an alternating electrical current such as a hairdryer. The current is located in the motor end, not the blower end, so it is the motor end you will be using to clear the smog.

Hold the motor end 6–12 inches from your body and move it over the whole of your body from top to toe. Move the hairdryer motor around your aura as though you are slowly cleaning a window. Pay particular attention to your head area and cover the whole of your auric field, even the soles of your feet. You may get the odd shiver, especially around your head. When this happens, it confirms that an energy shift is taking place and that it was needed.

It's easier if someone does this for you, as you won't be able to reach all parts of your back. It should only take a few minutes, and it is best to degauss late at night. Health kinesiologist practitioners say this process should be done a couple of times a week, but there are no hard and fast rules. If it works for you, use it whenever you feel the need.

What effect does geopathic stress have on sleep?

Geopathic stress is the belief that negative energies, or 'harmful earth rays', emanate from the earth and cause discomfort and ill health to organisms living directly above. If you have ever felt uneasy when you walked into a particular room or heard of people living in certain houses who are often ill, these can be indicators of geopathic stress.

Geopathic energy is described by some as etheric in nature, while others maintain it is natural radiation rising up through the earth, which then becomes distorted by subterranean running water, mineral concentrations, fault lines and underground cavities. These negative energies are said to result in geopathically stressed locations, which weaken the immune system and thus make one more susceptible to illness. Some say that while prolonged geopathic stress does not cause illness, it does lower the immune system and our ability to fight off viruses and bacteria.

Just as it is said that churches built on ley lines have a positive energy effect, so a house built on an area of geopathic stress could have a harmful effect on living organisms. Ley lines are positive energy lines that crisscross a land mass and historically have been used in many ancient cultures to site the location for spiritual monuments and temples.

Sceptics argue that geopathic stress is purely psychological and due to suggestion, but this does not explain how animals and plants respond to geopathic stress. Studies have shown that trees have stunted growth and do not bear fruit in geopathic hotspots. It is also said

☾ Sleep tip – mobile phone and EMF protection

Never leave your mobile phone by your bedside, even if it is switched off. Mobile phones give off the most EMFs at the time when they are switched on and off, so make a habit of turning yours on and off at arm's length. Better still, turn it on or off, then immediately put it down. Always avoid holding it close to your ear when switching on or off.

It is also prudent to buy an EMF protection device to attach to your mobile phone and computer equipment. These neat little chips are sometimes called mobile-phone protection chips, and they minimise the effects of EMF radiation.

that animals will seek to sleep in a geopathic-stress-free zone and that restless babies are sometimes responding to geopathic stress.

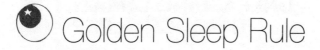 Golden Sleep Rule

6. Exercise!

Exercise regularly. Ideally take a little exercise each day –
do anything that gets your heart rate up. Regular exercise
will help you sleep well at night, so you absolutely must
get into the habit of moving your body and being active
on a daily basis.

Build regular exercise into your routine and work on
developing a mindset that loves exercising! Get into a
habit at least three times a week of indulging yourself
in specific exercise workouts, like working out at the
gym, practising yoga, playing tennis, cycling, jogging or
whatever works for you.

Chapter 11

UNLEASHING CREATIVITY THROUGH SLEEP

When we switch off our intellectual thought processes, we allow for greater access to our creative minds. It is often the busy chatter of the conscious mind that blocks our creativity. It has been said that people are at their most creative when logical, rational thought processes are suspended. This process obviously occurs when we sleep, but it also happens during hypnosis, meditation and daydreams.

The conscious part of the mind responsible for analysis, logic and practical thinking is in general terms a brain function of the left hemisphere. Most of our creative, emotional processes happen in the right hemisphere. The left hemisphere of the brain controls the right side of the body, and the right hemisphere controls the left-hand side of the body. Interestingly, at birth it is the other way around. The crossover only occurs when we reach around four years of age.

Sleep tip – lavender pillow

Sprinkle one or two drops of diluted lavender oil on your pillow just before you go to sleep at night. Lavender is often used as an aid to sleep and relaxation, and the subtle lavender aroma that you breathe in will relax and soothe you and help you sleep more soundly.

Creativity, sleep and dreaming

When you are switched off intellectually, you will naturally tap into your creative talents. This is why you will sometimes get stunningly brilliant ideas when you are daydreaming, as you are naturally connecting with the creativity that lies deep within your unconscious mind.

Hypnosis and meditation are great tools for creativity as they employ techniques to help you draw out your inner talents and inspiration. Many creative geniuses have known of this or had a natural ability to use this part of their mind at will. Mozart, for example, could hear a long, complex piece of music for the first time and then immediately play it note for note. He didn't have to think about it or analyse it, he could just do it, and from a very early age too. It was as though his unconscious creative processes were always open.

Another example is Paul McCartney, who woke up one morning in 1965 with the song 'Yesterday' in his head. He knew immediately it was a great song and at first couldn't believe that he had composed it in a dream. He played the first rendition of the song to other people to confirm that he hadn't plagiarised it. But sure enough, it was his own composition. The song went on to become the most frequently recorded song in the history of popular music, and the original Beatles' version was played on US radio alone more than six million times. As a budding songwriter, I long to wake up in the morning humming an original song of this calibre! So far no success, but I'm working on it! Paul also wrote the classic song 'Let It Be' after a dream about his mother, Mary, who had died ten years earlier.

Many other well-known historical figures have stated that their dreams were the inspiration behind their greatest achievements. Mary Shelley's enduring story *Frankenstein* came to fruition one morning after she literally dreamed up the central character. Charlie Chaplin would have a recording machine by the side of his bed as many of his ideas would come to him when he woke from sleeping. J. K. Rowling says she dreamed that she was the central character in *Harry Potter and the Deathly Hallows*, the final book, which helped her to complete the story.

Albert Einstein believed in the idea of switching off his intellectual mind to access his creative genius. He claimed that his theory of relativity came to him while he was in a trance state. He also gave us the quote 'Imagination is more important than knowledge. For knowledge is limited to all we now know and understand, while imagination embraces the entire world, and all there ever will be to know and understand.'

> ❝Keep true to the dreams of thy youth.❞
>
> *Friedrich von Schiller*
> (1759–1805)

Each of us has unlimited potential, and our truly great ideas lie deep inside our unconscious mind. This is where your real power and potential are hidden. The following technique will help you to connect with your creativity, which in turn will be the catalyst for new ideas and inspiration. It is a great technique if you are looking for a change in your career or some inspiration in general.

🌙 Creativity technique 🌙

This technique is ideal for getting new ideas and inspiration.

Before you go into the trance, imagine that you are going to draw new ideas from deep inside your unconscious mind into your conscious thoughts, as though you are going to open a door in your mind to an abundance of creativity and inspiration.

By now you will be familiar with going into a trance state and you can use any of the previous breathing and mind-calming techniques to get into a relaxed and centred state.

As you lie there in this stillness, feeling centred and very calm, connect with a part of you that is responsible for your creativity, the childlike, fun, creative part of you that is imaginative and carefree, the part that likes music and laughter. You can even imagine you are opening a door and entering a room that holds an unlimited source of creative inspiration. Take a moment to really feel this part of you and make a strong connection with it.

Now silently ask this creative part of you for guidance. Take a couple of minutes to do this. Ask it for ideas for new ventures. Don't force it; just allow the ideas to come. Sometimes you will get ideas and inspiration later.

Take five minutes here to be still and centred, and to allow your creative ideas to come forward. Imagine you are drawing ideas from a higher universal source where creativity flows in abundance.

After you have used this technique a few times, as an optional extra you may wish to add another stage to the technique.

Affirm to yourself that you will feel more creative and inspired in your daily life and that you can achieve many great things. State the following affirmations as a reality now in the present tense and, as always, supercharge them with your feelings:

I feel creative and inspired.

I have many new creative ideas.

I see opportunities all around me.

I believe in myself.

You may want to add your own present-tense phrases for creativity. When you state these phrases, draw the words inside you and really believe they are a reality. Put all your feelings into each phrase.

Now that you have opened up this channel, you may find new creative ideas come to you more often. It may be that this will manifest in getting new ideas out of the blue a day or two later. Practise this exercise often when you are looking for ideas or inspiration.

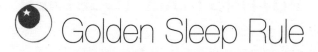 Golden Sleep Rule

7. Create the right bedroom environment.

Studies show that electromagnetic fields affect sleep patterns in a negative way. Televisions, hi-fi equipment, mobile or landline phones all emit strong electromagnetic fields and they are very detrimental to good-quality sleep.

Do not have any electrical items in your bedroom when you sleep. Your bedroom is for sleeping, and its environment should be conducive to sleep.

Chapter 12

PUTTING IT ALL TOGETHER

Your sleep diary

Now you are at the end of the programme, it would be worthwhile for you to begin a sleep diary so that you can learn more about your particular sleep patterns and see how they are improving. If you are sleeping through then congratulations and I do hope the quality of your life has improved. If you are still experiencing sleep disturbance or insomnia you may need to start the programme again and listen to the audio track more regularly.

To start your sleep diary keep a book and pen by your bedside and each morning note the following:

- The time you went to bed and the time you went to sleep.

- The total time you slept.

- How many times you woke up during the night and what you did. For example, 'continued to stay in bed with eyes closed', 'got up and stretched', 'had a glass of water' or 'meditated'.

- The quality of your night's sleep on a scale of one to ten, in which ten is deep, nourishing sleep, and one is fitful, restless sleep.

- The time you last ate and drank anything other than water, which ideally should be four hours before bedtime.

- How you felt before you went to sleep and when you woke up – for example, happiness, sadness, stress or anxiety.

- Remedies taken to help you sleep, amounts taken and times of consumption.

- What time you woke up and how you woke up. Was it naturally, with a daylight alarm clock, or did you wake suddenly?

- Any catnaps during the day.

After three months of using the accompanying audio download and the techniques in this book, notice how your sleep patterns change by comparing notes in your diary and reading your progression.

〗 Sleep tip – the ideal sleeping position

Some studies show that sleeping on the left side can cause your lungs, stomach and liver to press against your heart, causing stress. If you prefer to sleep on your side, try to do so on your right, not your left.

It is also interesting to know that sleeping on your stomach puts pressure on all of your internal organs, including your lungs, which can result in more shallow breathing. It can also exacerbate or result in a stiff neck and in upper-back problems.

How to measure how much sleep
you need

This is a good experiment to use at different times in your life as your personal sleep requirements will change with age. To test your sleep requirements conclusively, you will need a two-week period where you can go to bed at the same time each night and where you will not be governed by alarm clocks or any disturbances in the night or morning. This is so you can sleep and wake naturally without external prompts.

During this time you will need to make a note of approximately what time you fall asleep. You will need to let yourself wake naturally in the morning, then write down this time. If you then roll over and doze, this time does not count; it is when you wake up and become conscious that is your end point. You may well sleep more during the first few nights to repay your sleep debt, so ignore the results for the first few nights. You may notice that as you settle into a good sleeping pattern, you will have more energy in the day and feel more alert and refreshed.

Take the average sleep you get each night during the second week and see how this compares to the amount of sleep you actually get. If in your final week you are dropping off at midnight and waking around 8 a.m., then on average you need eight hours' sleep a night. If you are only getting six hours a night in your usual routine, you could be accumulating trouble for yourself. If you take lots of rest and relaxation at the weekend, or you take lots of holiday breaks where you repay this sleep debt, then you should be putting this right. If this is not the case because you are a workaholic or because of lifestyle commitments, you will need to make changes, as you cannot go on accumulating sleep debt without redemption.

If you don't make changes, your body may force you to. I have treated many burned-out executives in my practice. These are frequently people who are making a fortune in the City but working way too many hours in highly stressful environments. I often come across people with very successful careers who have become unable to function because of chronic insomnia, serious phobias or breakdowns. When you are out of balance, your brain and body have ways of forcing you to change.

☽ Sleep tip – bedtime reading

Do not read newspapers in bed at night or anything that may have a stimulating effect on your mind. Your aim should always be to calm your mind at bedtime, so if you do read anything, make sure it has a calming effect.

Coping with daily stress

The following section has a Reviewing the Day technique, which will help you sleep more peacefully. Before beginning your review of the day, it can help to view your life from a higher perspective as you lie in bed at night. By thinking along these lines, our daily stresses may feel less of a concern.

We all have busy lives that consume us and at times make us feel very important. But consider this: we are just one of six billion people inhabiting a tiny planet that is part of a small galaxy in a universe of billions of galaxies. To us, our illustrious life-giving sun is the one and only sun, but in reality it is just one of billions and billions of stars in an infinite universe that we can't even begin to comprehend.

Your world and the meanings of the events in your daily life come from your perspective. Nothing is absolute; it is just your interpretation. Whatever happens to us is neutral; nothing is for or against us in life, and things are only good or bad because we put our interpretation on them. Accept that the things that happen in your daily life, both good and bad, are opportunities to learn and grow.

If you worry about the terrible things that happen in the world – war, oppression, famine, manipulation, corruption, the evil that people do to others – think of this: the planet we live on is incredibly beautiful and has many wonders, but the light and beauty in our world also co-exist with dark forces.

If you believe in reincarnation, you and I chose to come on to this planet at a time of tremendous change so that we could experience the whole gamut of earthly existence – the good, the bad and everything in between. The world is as it should be and we are here to experience many of its extremes. Through our freewill we can make the world a better place if we choose to do good things and be of service to mankind. When we do this, it in turn helps our own evolution, as this is our reason for being here – to learn and evolve. There is nothing wrong with this world; it is perfect as it is. It is our school and eventual graduation.

I've heard many spiritual teachers say that the human experience is an incredibly heroic journey. In choosing as we did to incarnate into the earth plane at this time, our soul has embarked on a hazardous journey, but one with the potential for tremendous growth. With our freewill and willingness to learn, we can evolve spiritually and become more complete beings with the knowledge we acquire from our earthly experience.

Having a higher meaning in your life and viewing daily dramas from a bigger perspective will help bring you inner peace. It will empower you and help you to move forward with greater understanding. Make time to view the big picture.

🌙 Reviewing the Day 🌙 technique

This technique is particularly good to help you to de-stress if you have had a busy day and have lots on your mind.

Close your eyes and take a few slow, deep breaths. Allow your mind to become still and quiet for a couple of minutes. When your mind is blank, cast your thoughts back to the beginning of your day, when you first woke up. Then run through the events of your day from start to finish. Imagine all the things that happened sequentially and run it like a video in your mind. If there was anything unresolved, accept that a solution will come to you when the time is right. Make everything clear and bright as you visualise. Take as long as you need to do this.

Now imagine the events of your day from a higher perspective. You are one of billions of people on this planet, and you are doing the very best you can with the knowledge you have. Review the events of your day from this bigger, philosophical picture. Look at the good and bad events of your day as opportunities for you to learn. Accept that every experience you have is valuable and that life is a series of ups and downs, in the same way that nature and the seasons ebb and flow. Imagine yourself on your journey riding the highs and lows of life, and enjoying the journey as a whole, becoming wiser from every small experience.

Then, when you are finished, imagine you are letting it all go, so that you feel detached from the events of your day. Imagine the day as a whole drifting away so that your mind becomes still and quiet.

You may even continue your deep breathing as you let go of everything – this will help you to relax deeply and go to sleep more easily. Imagine you are breathing away any cares or worries.

This technique can help you unwind and sleep more deeply, as you are letting go of the mental stresses that keep you awake.

Sleep in peace

Congratulations on reaching the end of the book. You are now armed with all the tools you need to help you sleep well at night. The key to my programme is to continue to use the techniques and tips that are most relevant to your sleep problem.

You may find that the positive changes are instant or it may be that you move into new healthy sleep patterns over a period of time. Many people who use my sleep audio download are able to sleep well using the audio alone but with the programme you have a failsafe and holistic solution, a solution that works, covering a wide range of sleep problems.

By taking action, following the simple steps and using the recording each night you are empowering yourself on a deep level. Your mind and body will naturally adapt so that sleeping soundly becomes second nature to you. You will wake refreshed and ready to face the day.

So, welcome to the rest of your life and may you sleep well each and every night!

Glenn

FURTHER RESOURCES

Further Reading

Dave Elman, *Hypnotherapy* (Westwood Publishing Company, 1984) A classic on hypnosis first published in 1960 and still very relevant.

Janey Lee Grace, *Imperfectly Natural Woman: Getting Life Right the Natural Way* (Crown House Publishing, 2005) A fabulous book on holistic living from a writer with a down-to-earth approach.

Glenn Harrold, *Look Young, Live Longer* (Orion, 2019) A book with hypnosis audio that will help you feel young again.

Glenn Harrold, *Lose Weight Now!* (Orion, 2019) A book with hypnosis audio that will help you take control of your weight.

Glenn Harrold, *De-stress Your Life* (Orion, 2019) A book with hypnosis audio that will help you to de-stress all areas of your life.

Glenn Harrold, *The Answer* (Orion, 2013) A book that will show you how to find health, wealth and true happiness.

Glenn Harrold, *Create Wealth and Abundance* (Diviniti
   Publishing, 2005) A book and hypnosis CD that will help
   you create financial abundance.

Patrick Holford, *New Optimum Nutrition Bible: the Book You Have
   to Read If You Care About Your Health* (Piatkus Books, 2004)

Karen Kingston, *Clear Your Clutter with Feng Shui: Space-clearing
   Can Change Your Life* (Piatkus Books, 1998)

Felicity Lawrence, *Not on the Label* (Penguin, 2004) An
   eye-opening book on the food industry. A must-read!

Jason Vale, *The Juice Master: Turbo-charge Your Life in 14 Days*
   (HarperCollins, 2005) Common-sense advice on healthy
   eating with many valuable tips. Includes an excellent
   detox plan.

Jason Vale, *Chocolate Busters: the Easy Way to Kick Your Addiction*
   (HarperCollins, 2005) Will help you break the chocolate
   habit for ever.

Further Viewing

Glenn Harrold, *Lose Weight Now* (Diviniti Publishing, 2007)
A 40-minute hypnotherapy DVD to help you lose weight.
   Includes subliminal imagery.

Glenn Harrold, *Complete Relaxation* (Diviniti Publishing, 2007)
A 40-minute relaxation hypnotherapy DVD. Includes
   subliminal imagery.

Shiva Rea: Yoga Shakti (Gemini Sun, 2004)
A professional DVD for a complete yoga workout.

Further Listening

Glenn Harrold, *Relax and Sleep Well* (free app)

Glenn Harrold, *Ultimate Hypnosis* (free app)

Glenn Harrold, *Complete Relaxation* (Diviniti Publishing, 1999)

Glenn Harrold, *Lose Weight Now* (Diviniti Publishing, 1999)

Finding a well-qualified hypnotherapist in the UK

When seeking out a hypnotherapist for a one-to-one session, it is advisable to contact a few in your area. The organisation I trained with, the **British Society of Clinical Hypnosis** (BSCH), has a register of qualified hypnotherapists throughout the UK. The website address is www.bsch.org.uk.

The training is of the highest standard, although the quality of individual therapists can vary. I suggest you call a few locally and find someone with whom you feel comfortable. Good therapy is all about the dynamic between the therapist and client. Finding a therapist who inspires you and who can get to the root of your problem is the key.

The **Association for Professional Hypnosis and Psychotherapy** (APHP) is another useful body to contact. It is made up of well-qualified therapists who have formed their own group and have hand-picked other therapists to join them. So, on the whole, they should be good. The website address is www.aphp.co.uk, and the phone number is 01702 347 691.

UK hypnotherapy college courses

If you are interested in training to become a hypnotherapist, the **London College of Clinical Hypnosis** is one of the biggest and best in the UK. Their courses are comprehensive and offer in-depth training in the art of hypnotherapy.

> The London College of Clinical Hypnosis
> 7 Bury Place
> London WC1A 2LA
> Telephone: +44 (0)020 3603 8535
> Website: www.lcchinternational.co.uk
> Email: info@lcchinternational.co.uk

Qualifying via the London College means you are automatically eligible for membership of the British Society of Clinical Hypnosis. The BSCH has centres all over the UK, and the organisation ensures that training is of a high standard. The best way to learn and succeed in hypnotherapy is in a classroom setting with comprehensive training.

More about me

For an up-to-date list of my titles, contact:

Diviniti Publishing Ltd
Unit 1 Bourne Enterprise Centre
Wrotham Road
Borough Green
Kent TN15 8DG
Telephone: 01732 882 057
Email: sales@hypnosisaudio.com

My CDs and downloads can be purchased from www.hypnosisaudio.com, and my personal website is www.glennharrold.com.